The complete New Mediterranean Diet Cookbook For Beginners 2024:

Featuring Over 200 Delicious, Easy and Stress Free Recipes With 30 Day Meal Plan

Katherine Miller

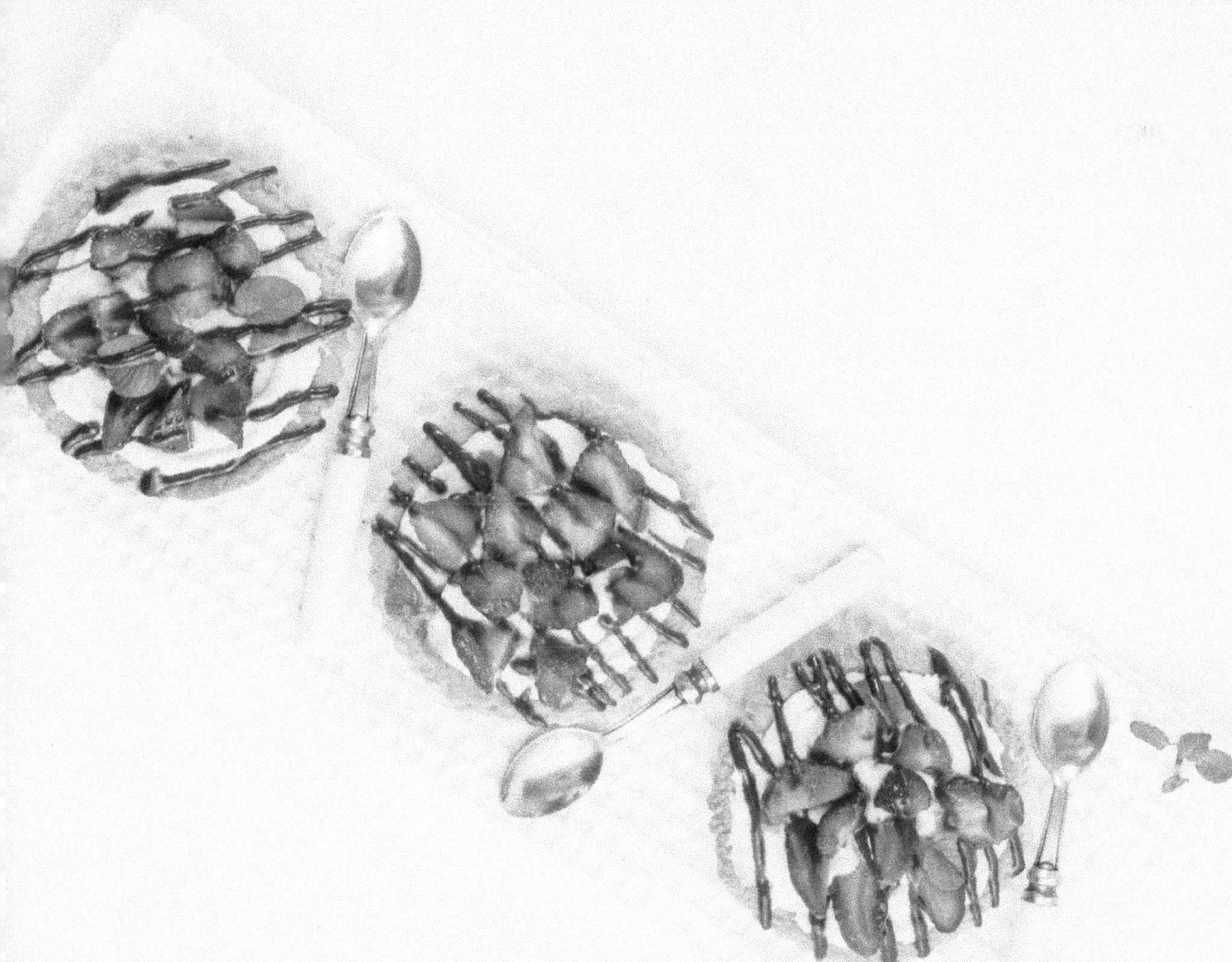

Copyright © 2023 by Katherine Miller

ISBN: 978-1-961902-81-7

This book is published by **Litbooks** Publishers.

Paperback Edition

First Edition: 2023

Table of Contents

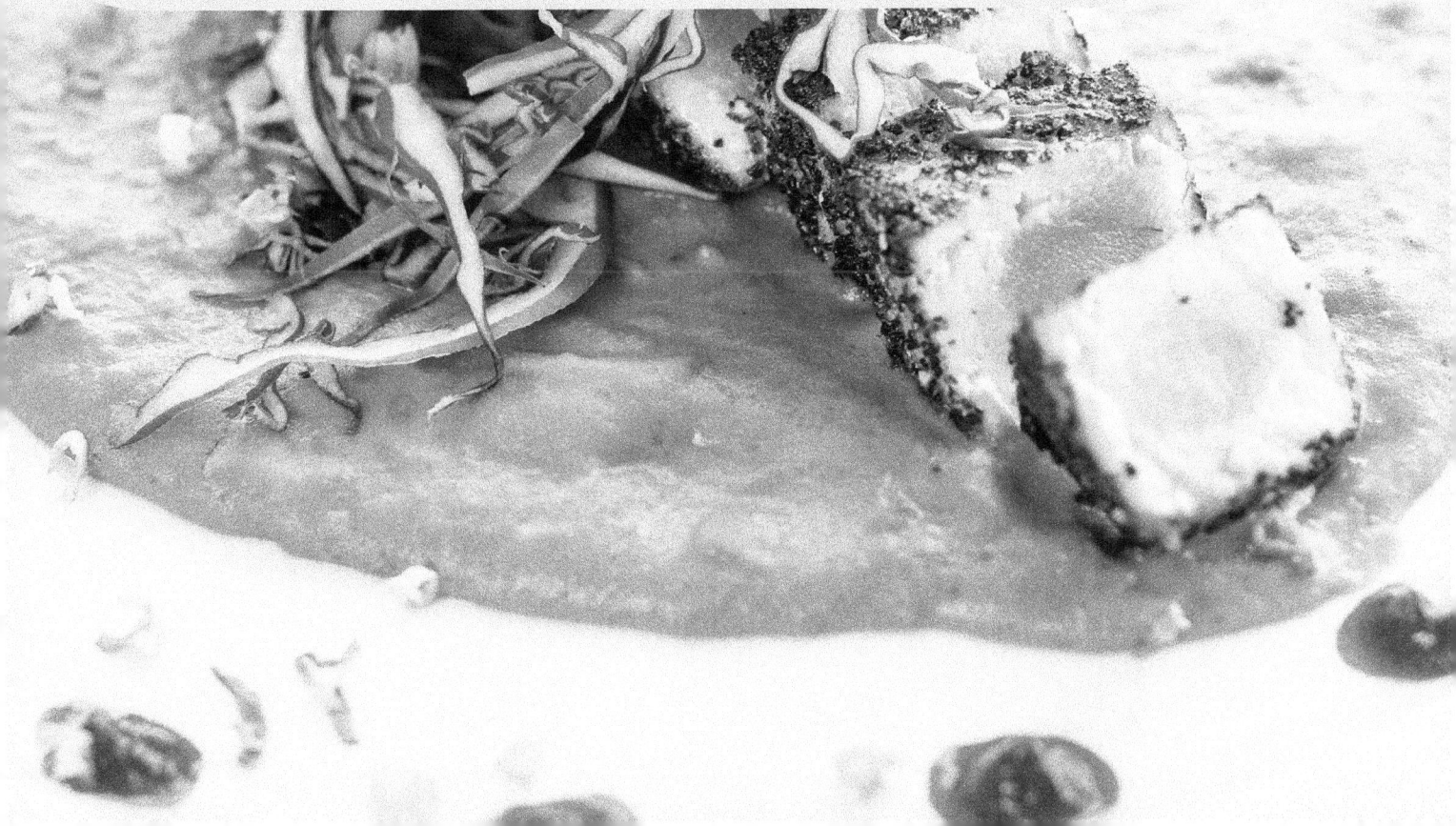

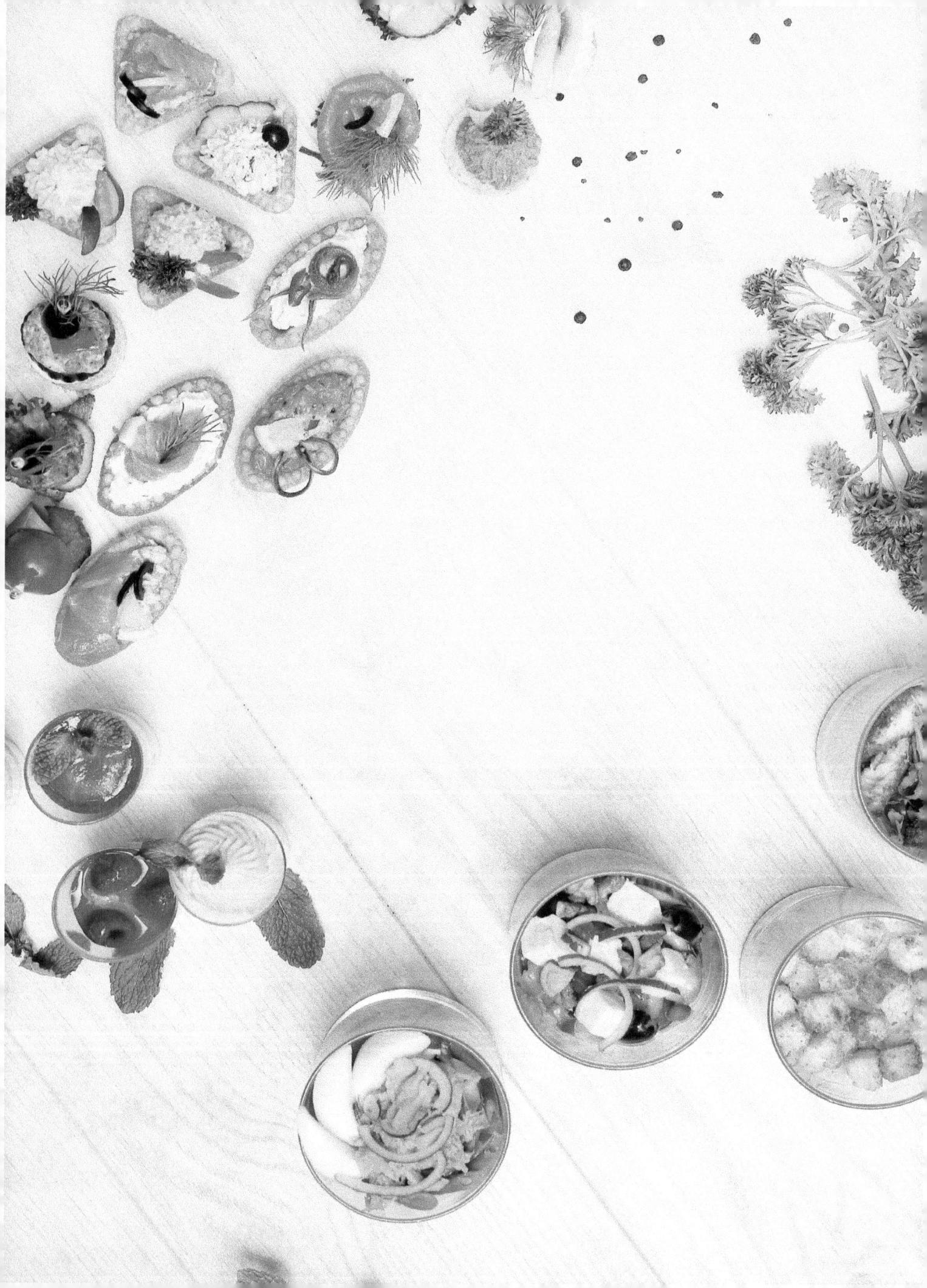

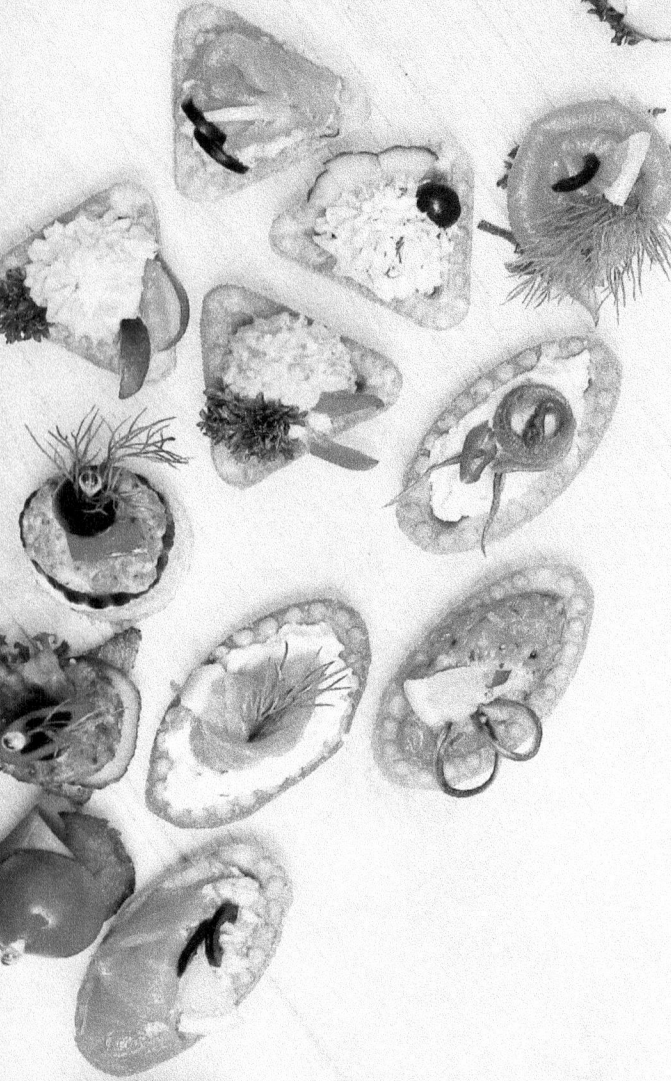

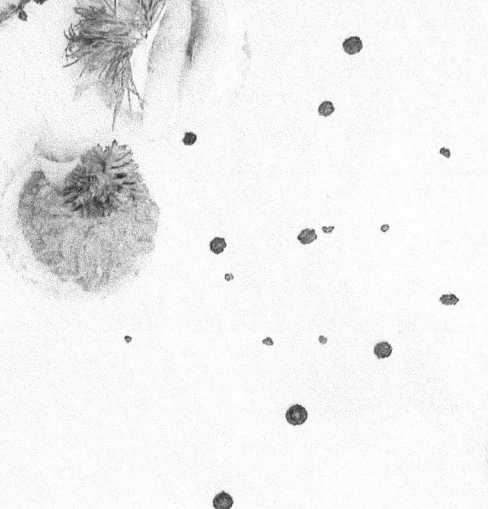

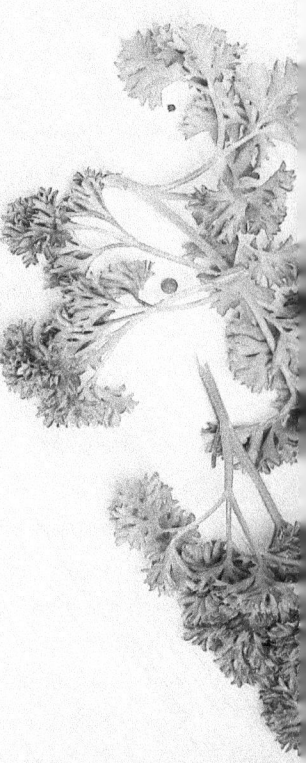

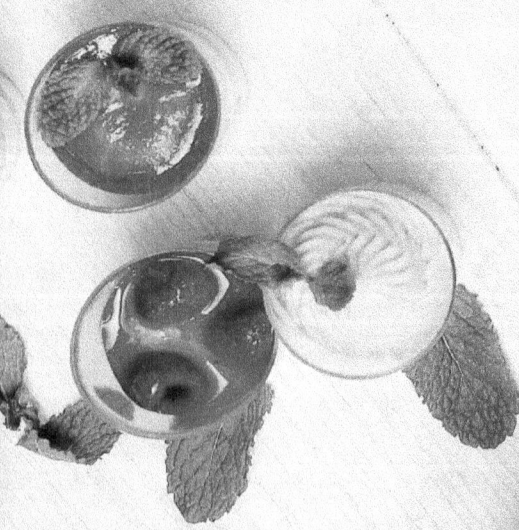

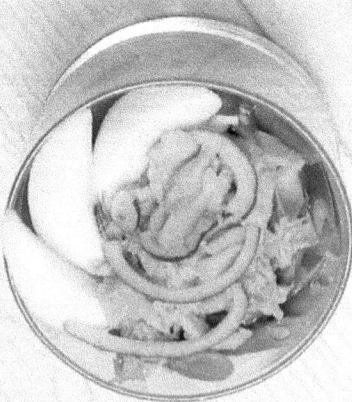

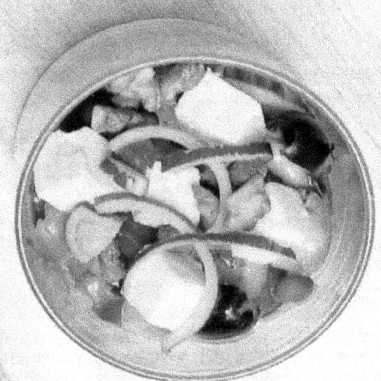

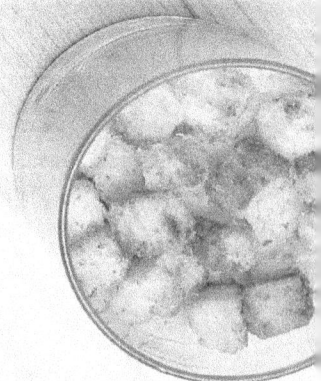

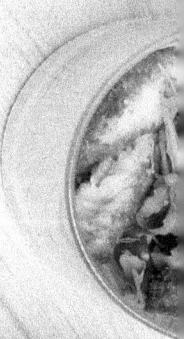

Introduction

Discover the vibrant and diverse culinary world that encircles the Mediterranean Sea, a region rich in culture and flavors. From the sun-kissed coasts of Italy, France, and Spain to the ancient lands of Greece, Turkey, Israel, and beyond, and down to the North African shores of Egypt, Tunisia, and Morocco, the Mediterranean diet offers a tapestry of tastes and traditions.

In this introduction to the "New Mediterranean Diet for Beginners," we delve into the heart of what makes this diet universally appealing and incredibly healthy. It's not about a singular, homogenized cuisine, but rather the shared principles that these varied cultures embrace. Fresh vegetables and fruits, a bounty of beans and lentils, wholesome whole grains, a preference for seafood over meat and poultry, and the liberal use of heart-healthy olive oil form the cornerstone of the Mediterranean way of eating.

This book is more than just a collection of recipes; it's an invitation to experience the essence of the Mediterranean lifestyle. Each recipe is a celebration of the common dietary threads that weave through this diverse region. Whether you're a beginner in the world of Mediterranean cooking or looking to expand your culinary horizons, this book offers a simple, yet compelling, gateway to healthier eating and a flavorful journey through the Mediterranean's rich culinary landscape. Embark on this delicious adventure and embrace the Mediterranean way of life, one plate at a time.

The Mediterranean Diet

At its core, the Mediterranean diet isn't just about what's on your plate, but rather a lifestyle that emphasizes balance, diversity, and wholesomeness; Here are some nutritional ingredients;

1. **Olive Oil:** Not just any oil, but the golden nectar of the Mediterranean. It's the backbone of every dish, offering both sumptuous flavors and impressive health benefits.

2. **Fresh Produce:** Think bright red tomatoes, sun-kissed peppers, and crunchy cucumbers. The region's sun ensures an abundance of flavorful and nutrient-rich veggies.

3. **Seafood:** Given the vast coastline, it's no wonder fish is a staple. From sardines to salmon, the Mediterranean Sea offers a mixture of heart-healthy options.

4. **Whole Grains:** Farro, bulgur, and couscous are among the many grains that give Mediterranean dishes their comforting textures.

5. **Legumes:** Beans, lentils, and chickpeas are not only a protein source but also lend themselves to countless stews and salads.

6. **Herbs & Spices:** Rosemary, thyme, oregano, and saffron are just a pinch of the flavorful world of the Mediterranean.

It's a Lifestyle, Not Just a Diet

The Mediterranean diet isn't just about food. It's also about how you consume it. It consists of;
1. Social Dining: Sharing meals with family and friends is more than a tradition; it's a celebration of life.
2. Mindful Eating: Take the time to savor every bite, enjoying the array of flavors and textures.
3. Active Living: Walk through olive groves, dance during local festivals, or simply take a leisurely stroll after dinner. Movement is as essential as what you eat.

Embrace a Healthy Lifestyle

The Mediterranean diet isn't famous just because it's delicious. Its fame also stems from its profound health benefits.

1. **Heart's Best Friend:** With unsaturated fats, fresh produce, and limited red meat, this diet keeps the heart pumping and smiling.

2. **Brain Booster:** Ingredients rich in antioxidants and omega-3s, like olive oil and fish, pave the way for a sharp mind.

3. **Weight Wellness:** With its emphasis on natural and whole foods, it's a sustainable way to maintain a healthy weight.

Simple, Unforgettable Meals

It's not about extravagant dishes but simplicity that steals the show.

1. **Greek Salad:** Fresh tomatoes, cucumbers, and feta cheese drizzled with olive oil – a symphony of freshness.

2. **Hummus:** This chickpea dip, blended with tahini and olive oil, is a testament to how basic ingredients can create magic.

3. **Grilled Fish:** Just a squeeze of lemon, a sprinkle of herbs, and the natural flavors of the sea come alive.

What to Expect with a Mediterranean Diet?

The Mediterranean diet isn't just a diet; it's a celebration of life. Embarking on this journey means more than just changing what's on your plate. Here's what you can look forward to:

1. **A Colorful Plate**: First and foremost, expect a splash of vibrant colors every mealtime. Think deep green olives, ruby-red tomatoes, sunny-yellow peppers, and the azure blue of the sea mirrored in fresh fish.

2. **Flavor, Not Fads**: This isn't a 'lose 10 pounds in 10 days' kind of diet. The Mediterranean way is about savoring every bite, enjoying a mix of herbs, fresh ingredients, and diverse textures. It's a timeless approach, rather than a fleeting trend.

3. **Friendship over Forks**: Meals are shared moments. In the Mediterranean, dining is a communal activity. Expect laughter, stories, and moments of connection.

4. **Move with Joy**: It's not all about food. This lifestyle embraces daily physical activity, whether it's a breezy walk along the beach or a spirited dance under the stars.

5. **Less Is More**: Here, meat plays a guest role, not the main act. Expect more plant-based meals, with meat sprinkled in as a treat, rather than the centerpiece.

6. **Sea's the Day**: Fish, particularly oily ones like sardines and salmon, will make regular appearances on your plate, bringing with them a wealth of omega-3s.

7. **Liquid Gold**: Olive oil will become your kitchen's best friend. Not only does it elevate the taste of dishes, but it's also packed with heart-healthy fats.

8. **Wine and Dine**: If you enjoy a glass of wine, you'll appreciate that it's a part of this diet – in moderation, of course. A glass with dinner is customary, emphasizing the pleasure of dining rather than drinking to excess.

9. **Sweets, naturally**: Desserts aren't forbidden, but they're often fruit-based. Think juicy grapes, sweet figs, or honey-drizzled melons. For those special occasions, pastries and cakes do make an appearance, but they're enjoyed mindfully and in moderation.

10. **Endless Possibilities**: With such a vast range of ingredients and flavors, there's no room for monotony. Every meal is a new opportunity to experiment, creating a lifelong romance with food.

Embracing the Mediterranean diet is like diving into a deep blue sea of flavor, health, and joy. It's more than just eating; it's living in full color.

Next we take a look at the Mediterranean food pyramid and jump right into the recipe.

Drawing inspiration from the Mediterranean Diet Pyramid, this book is a captivating guide to a heart-healthy and flavorful lifestyle. Rooted in the Harvard School of Public Health and Oldways' collaborative efforts, it reflects the dietary wisdom from Ancel Keys' renowned Seven Countries Study.

Emphasizing fruits, vegetables, grains, and olive oil, with moderate consumption of fish, poultry, and dairy, and minimal intake of meats and sweets, these recipes are designed to tantalize your taste buds while promoting overall well-being.

Experience a diet celebrated for its cardiovascular benefits and links to improved cognitive function, weight management, and long-term health. Dive into this culinary adventure, where each recipe brings the vibrant, satisfying essence of the Mediterranean right into your kitchen.

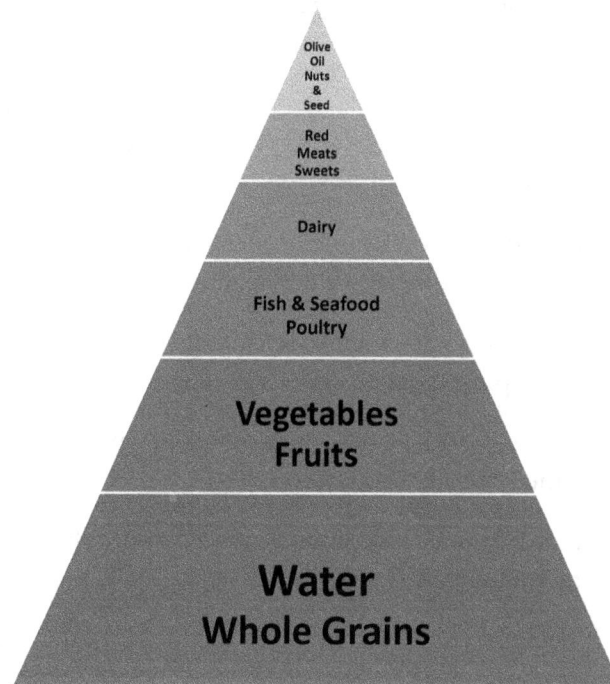

Olive
Oil
Nuts
&
Seed

Red
Meats
Sweets

Dairy

Fish & Seafood
Poultry

Vegetables
Fruits

Water
Whole Grains

Breakdown of the Mediterranean Food Pyramid:
1. Base Layer: Daily Essentials (50%)
- **Water**: Drink water regularly for hydration and overall health.

- **Whole Grains**: Foods like barley, bulgur, and farro are energy sources. Include them in daily meals.

2. Second Layer: Fruits & Vegetables (30%)
- **Vegetables**: Vegetables provide essential vitamins, antioxidants, and fiber. Aim to fill half your plate with various vegetables.

- **Fruits**: Fruits offer natural sugars, vitamins, and fiber. Eat them daily, either as snacks or desserts.

3. Third Layer: Proteins (10%)
- **Fish & Seafood**: Focus on fish for lean protein and omega-3s. Try to eat fish at least twice a week.

- **Poultry**: Opt for chicken or turkey as a lean protein source, and eat it in moderation.

4. Fourth Layer: Dairy (7%)
- **Dairy**: Foods like yogurt and cheese are sources of calcium and beneficial bacteria. Use them moderately to complement meals.

5. Fifth Layer: Treats (2%)

- **Red Meats**: While flavorful, red meats are higher in saturated fats. Consume them sparingly.

- **Sweets**: Enjoy sweet treats occasionally, not daily.

Top of the Pyramid: Fats (1%)

- **Olive Oil, Nuts, and Seeds**: These provide good fats essential for the body. Olive oil should be the main cooking and dressing fat.

Lifestyle Recommendations:

- **Physical Activity**: Regular exercise or activity is beneficial.

- **Social Interaction**: Sharing meals with friends and family is essential in the Mediterranean lifestyle.

Getting Started
Creating a Mediterranean Table: A Guide to Healthier, Flavorful Eating

1. **Rethink Your Plate:** Shift to a Mediterranean mindset where meals feature smaller, balanced portions of vegetables, grains, and proteins. Think 'small plates' rather than a single main dish, creating a more diverse and satisfying dining experience.

2. **Moderation is Essential:** Embrace smaller portion sizes characteristic of the Mediterranean diet. Our recipes are designed to reflect this philosophy, focusing on appropriate amounts of various dishes for a complete meal.

3. **Seasonal and Fresh:** Prioritize vegetables and fruits daily, choosing seasonal and local produce for the freshest flavors. Utilize reliable substitutes like jarred or frozen options when fresh isn't available.

4. **Protein Balance:** Incorporate more beans, lentils, nuts, and whole grains for protein, while reducing red meat consumption. Enjoy fish and seafood regularly for their health benefits and variety.

5. **Desserts with a Twist:** End your meals with fresh fruits or carefully chosen sweets, made healthier in our recipes with smart substitutions like olive oil. Embrace the joy of balanced, satisfying desserts.

Dive into this culinary adventure, where each recipe offers a taste of the vibrant Mediterranean lifestyle. Embrace variety, balance, and the joy of fresh, healthy eating. Let our guide lead you to a table brimming with flavor and nourishment. Start your journey to a healthier, more flavorful life today!

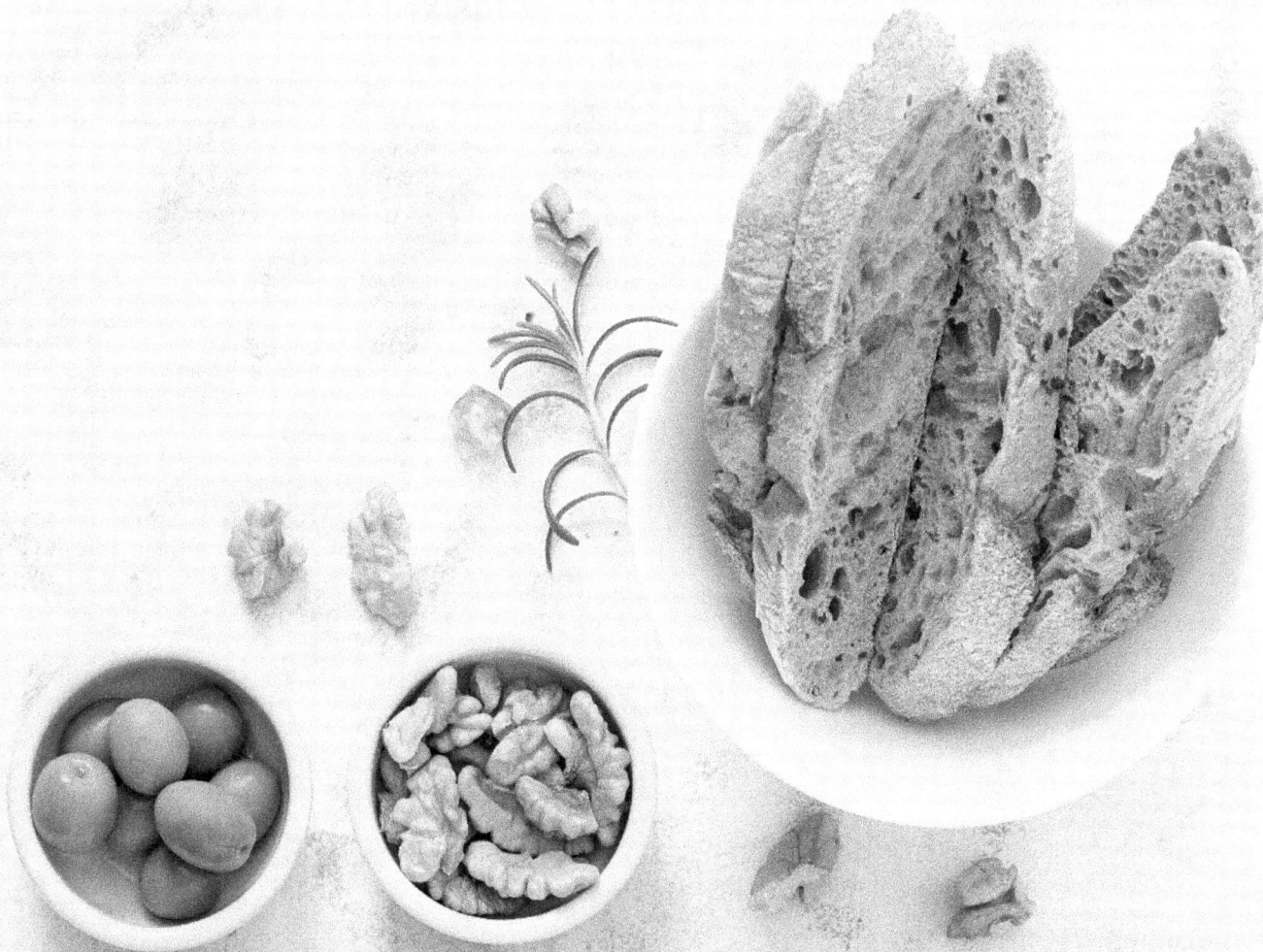

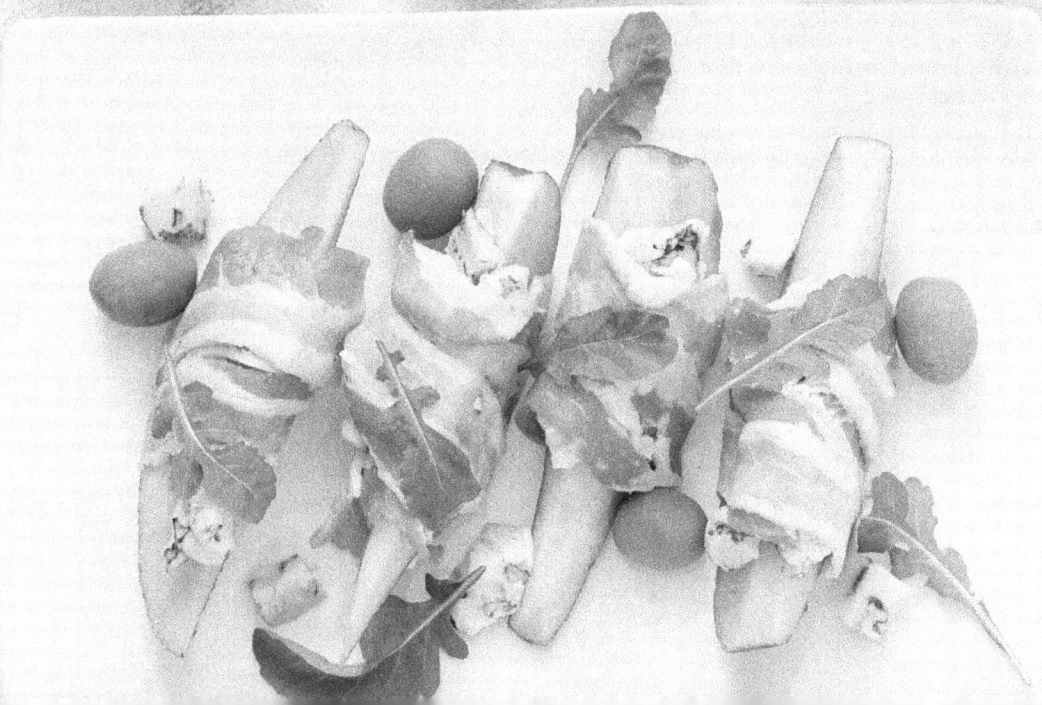

1. Eggs with Zucchini Noodles

Preparation time: 10min / Cooking time: 15min / Servings: 2
Ingredients:

- 3 Zucchini spiralized into noodles
- 2 Tbsp Olive Oil
- 1 Cup Cherry Tomatoes halved
- Sea salt and freshly ground black pepper, to taste
- 4 Eggs
- 1 Avocado halved and thinly sliced
- ¼ Cup Crumbled Feta Cheese
- 1 Tbsp Fresh Chopped Parsley

Directions:

- Preheat the oven to 350°F. Lightly spray a baking sheet with cooking spray.
- In a large bowl, toss the zucchini noodles, cherry tomatoes and olive oil to combine. Season with salt and pepper to your taste.
- Divide into 4 even portions on your baking sheet and shape each into a nest, then gently crack an egg in the center of each one.
- Bake until the eggs are set, 8-12 minutes. Top with avocado slices, crumbled cheese, and parsley. Enjoy!

Nutrition Per Serving: calories 262kcal | Protein 10g | carbs 11g | fat 21g | fiber 5g

2. Avocado Toast with Poached Egg and Cherry Tomatoes

Preparation Time: 10 mins | Cooking Time: 10mins | Servings: 2
Ingredients:

- 2 slices of whole-grain bread
- 1 ripe avocado
- 2 large eggs
- 1 cup cherry tomatoes, halved
- 1 tablespoonful olive oil
- Salt and black pepper to taste
- Optional toppings: chopped parsley, red pepper flakes, crumbled feta cheese

Directions:

- Toast the bread slices until golden brown.
- While the bread is toasting, prepare the avocado by cutting it in half, removing the pit and scooping out the flesh into a bowl. Mash the avocado with a fork until it reaches your desired consistency.
- In a separate pan, heat up the olive oil over medium heat. Add the halved cherry tomatoes and sauté for about 3-4 minutes, until they start to soften.
- Fill a small saucepan with water and bring it to a gentle simmer. Crack each egg into a separate ramekin or small bowl. Carefully lower the eggs into the simmering water and cook for about 3 minutes, until the whites are set and the yolks are still runny.
- Spread the mashed avocado evenly on the two slices of toasted bread. Top each slice with the sautéed cherry tomatoes.
- Using a slotted spoon, carefully remove each poached egg from the water and place one on top of each slice of bread.
- Sprinkle with salt and black pepper to taste. Add any optional toppings, such as chopped parsley, red pepper flakes or crumbled feta cheese.

Nutrition Per Serving: Calories: 485 | Total fat: 32g | Saturated fat: 6g | Cholesterol: 186mg | Sodium: 298mg | Total Carbohydrates: 36g | Dietary fiber: 12g | Sugars: 4g | Protein: 17g

3. Ham 'N Cheese Scrambled Eggs

Prep Time 15 min | Total Time 25 min
Ingredients:

- 3 tbsp Land O Lakes® Butter
- 1 small (1/2 cup of) onion, chopped
- 1 small (1/2 cup of) green bell pepper, chopped
- 1 1/2 cup of (cubed 1/2-inch) cooked ham
- 12 large Land O Lakes® Eggs
- 3 tbsp water
- 1 cup of shredded Cheddar cheese
- Salt, if desired
- Pepper, if desired

Direction:

- In the 12-inch nonstick skillet, melt butter over medium-high heat until it sizzles, then add onion and green pepper. Cooks 3-4 minutes, stirring occasionally, or until vegetables are crisp-tender. Cook for another 2-3 minutes, or until the ham is cooked through. Reduce to a medium heat environment.
- In a mixing cup of, whisk together the eggs and the water. In a skillet, crack eggs and pour them over the vegetables. Cook 3-4 minutes or until almost set, gently raising and stirring with spatula to allow uncooked portion to flow underneath.
- Add cheese and season with salts and pepper, if necessary. Cover and switch off the sun. Allow to sits for 2 to 3 minutes.

4. Fried Eggs with Smoked Salmon and Lemon Cream

Preparation Time: 20 minutes | serves: 2
Ingredients:

- 4 Eggs
- 2 oz Smoked salmon
- 2 tbsp Sour cream
- 1 tbsp Butter
- 1 Chives, stalk
- 3/4 tsp Lemon juice
- 1/4 tbsp Lemon peel
- 1/4 tsp Cumin leaves

Directions

- In a small bowl, mix the sour cream, lemon juice, zest, and chopped cumin leaves. Mix well.
- In another bowl, lightly beat the eggs, salt, and pepper.
- Melt the butter in a frying pan over medium heat. Add chopped spring onions and pass for 1 minute.
- Then pour the eggs and cook, stirring constantly, for 1 minute. Arrange on 2 plates.
- Top with thinly sliced fish and sprinkle with lemon cream.

Nutrition per serving: Calories: 192 Kcal | Fat: 15.3 g. | Protein: 11.7 g. | Carbs: 1.2 g

5. Avocado Breakfast Scramble

Number of servings: 1
Ingredients:

- 2 large eggs
- ½ avocado, peeled, pitted, sliced
- Juice of ½ lime
- ½ tablespoon butter, cubed
- Freshly cracked pepper to taste
- A small handful of cherry or grape tomatoes, halved
- Salt to taste

Directions:

- Add eggs, salt, and butter to a pan. Place the pan over medium-low heat. Stir often and cook until the eggs are soft-cooked.
- Transfer the scrambled eggs to a plate. Scatter avocado and tomatoes over the eggs. Sprinkle salt, pepper, and lime juice on top and serve.

Nutrition per serving: Calories: 254 | Fat: 17.15g | Carbohydrates: 16.05g | Fiber: 3.44g | Protein: 10.99g

6. Blueberry Coffee Breakfast Smoothie

Number of servings: 1
Ingredients:

- ½ cup rolled oats
- 1 teaspoon instant coffee
- ½ cup almond milk
- ½ cup fresh blueberries
- 3 dates, pitted

Directions:
1. Place oats, coffee, almond milk, blueberries, and dates in a blender.
2. Blend until very smooth.
3. Pour into a glass and serve.

Nutrition Per Serving: Calories – 199 | Fat – 3 g | Carbohydrate – 41 g | Fiber – 5 g | Protein – 4 g

7. Mixed Berry Oatmeal

Preparation time: 1 min / Cooking time: 5 min / Servings: 2
Ingredients:

- 1 cup Bob's Red Mill Quick Cooking Rolled Oats
- 1 cup mixed berries - blueberries, strawberries, blackberries, whatever you wish
- 1 tbsp honey
- 2 tsp brown sugar, divided

Directions:

- Cook the oats according to package directions.
- While the oats are cooking, combine the berries and honey in a saucepan set over medium heat on the stove. Cook until the fruit releases its juices -- about 3-5 minutes. Remove from heat.
- Divide the oatmeal between two bowls. Top each with 1 teaspoon of brown sugar, and 1/2 of the berry mixture. -Enjoy!

Nutrition Per Serving: calories 248kcal |protein 6g |carbs 51g | fat 3g | fiber 8g

8. Breakfast Granola

Preparation Time: 5 minutes | Cooking Time: 5 minutes| Serving: 6
Ingredients:

- ½ cup oats
- 1 teaspoon ground cinnamon
- 1/3 cup sliced almonds
- 2 tablespoons shredded coconut
- 2 tablespoons sunflower seeds
- 1 tablespoon flax seeds
- 1 teaspoon coconut oil
- 2 tablespoons honey

Directions

- Take a medium bowl, place all the ingredients in it and then stir until well mixed.
- Take a skillet pan, place it over medium heat, add the granola mixture and then cook for 3 to 5 minutes until toasted.
- Meal Prep: Let the granola cool completely, place it in an air-tight jar and then seal it.
- When ready to eat, one-sixth place portion of the granola in a bowl, add milk, top with fruit slices, and then serve.

Nutrition per Serving: Calories: 120 Cal | Total Fats: 7 g | Saturated Fat: 2 g | Carbohydrate: 14 g | Sugar: 7 g | Fiber: 2 g | Protein: 3 g

9. Mediterranean Breakfast Board

Preparation Time: 30 mins | Total Time: 30 minutes
Ingredients

- 1 Falafel Recipe
- 1 Classic Hummus Recipe
- 1 Baba Ganoush Recipe
- Feta cheese
- 1 Tabouli Recipe
- 1 to 2 tomatoes, sliced
- 1 English cucumber, sliced
- 6 to 7 Radish, halved or sliced
- Assorted olives
- Marinated artichokes or mushrooms
- Early Harvest EVOO and Za'atar to dip
- Pita Bread, sliced into quarters
- Grapes (palette cleanser)
- Fresh herbs for garnish

Directions

- Note: For quick and easy assembly, make the majority of these ahead of time. See the notes for further information.
- Make the falafel according to the directions on the package. To soak the chickpeas, you'll need to start at least the night before. For working ahead, see the notes below. (Falafel can also be purchased at a Middle Eastern market.)
- Make the hummus and baba ganoush according to the directions in this recipe. Both of these may be made the night before and stored in the refrigerator. To spice things up, try roasted garlic hummus or roasted red pepper hummus.

- Using this recipe, slice feta cheese or make Labneh ahead of time.
- To make tabouli, follow this recipe. It's possible to make it ahead of time and keep it refrigerated in glass containers with tight lids.
- Place a hummus, baba ganoush, olive oil, za'atar, and tabouli in bowls to make the Mediterranean breakfast board. To create a focal point, place the biggest bowl in the center of a big wooden board or platter.
- If desired, garnish with fresh herbs and grapes.

10. Scrambled Eggs with Bell Peppers, Onions, and Cheddar Cheese

Preparation time: 15 minutes | Cooking Time: 10mins | Servings: 2
Ingredients:
- 4 eggs
- 1/2 red bell pepper, diced
- 1/2 green bell pepper, diced
- 1/4 onion, diced
- 1/2 cup shredded cheddar cheese
- 2 tablespoonfuls olive oil
- Salt and pepper to taste
- Fresh parsley for garnish

Directions:
- Heat 1 tablespoonful of olive oil in a non-stick pan over medium heat.
- Add the diced bell peppers and onions to the pan and sauté for 3-4 minutes until they start to soften.
- In a separate bowl, beat the eggs with salt and pepper.
- Add the beaten eggs to the pan with the bell peppers and onions and scramble until the eggs are fully cooked.
- Sprinkle shredded cheddar cheese over the eggs and let it melt.
- Divide the scrambled eggs onto two plates, garnish with fresh parsley, and serve.

Nutrition per Serving: Calories: 300 | Fat: 22g | Protein: 20g | Carbohydrates: 7g | Fiber: 2g

11. Berry Chia Pudding

Number of servings: 4
Ingredients:
- 3 ½ cups blackberries or raspberries or diced mangoes, divided
- ½ cup chia seeds
- 1 ½ teaspoons vanilla extract
- ½ cup granola
- 2 cups unsweetened almond milk or milk choice
- 2 tablespoons maple syrup
- 1 cup whole-milk plain Greek yogurt

Directions:
- Blend together 2 ½ cups berries and milk in a blender until very smooth.
- Pour into a bowl. Add chia seeds, vanilla, and maple syrup and stir. Cover the bowl with cling wrap and chill overnight. This can last for three days.

- To assemble: Take four glasses. Layer with chia pudding, remaining berries and yogurt in whatever manner you desire.
- Top each glass with two tablespoons granola and serve.

Nutrition per serving: One glass
Calories: 343 | Fat: 15.4 g | Carbohydrates: 39.4 g | Fiber: 14.9 g | Protein: 13.8 g'

12. Mediterranean Tofu Scramble

Number of servings: 4
Ingredients:
- 2 tablespoons olive oil
- Himalayan pink salt to taste
- ½ cup sundried tomatoes in oil, cut into strips
- Chopped chives, to garnish
- 20 ounces firm tofu, crumbled
- 2 teaspoons mild curry powder
- 2/3 cup green olives pitted, sliced into rings

Directions:
- Pour oil into a nonstick pan and heat over medium-high flame. Once the oil is hot, add tofu. Stir in curry powder and Himalayan pink salt.
- Cook for about 5 minutes, stirring frequently.
- Add sundried tomatoes and olives and heat thoroughly

13. Baked Eggs with Pesto

Preparation Time: 25 minutes | serves: 4
Ingredients:
- 8 Egg
- 1/4 glass
- 2 fl. oz Cream 35%
- 2 oz Butter
- 2 tbsp Pesto sauce
- Black ground pepper, to taste

Directions:
- Take small baking tins and grease them inside with butter. In each form, break into 2 eggs, trying not to damage the shell of the yolk. Salt, pepper, and add a little cream.
- Bake the eggs in the oven for 16-20 minutes at 160 degrees. Wait until the cream thickens, and the proteins become opaque, and remove from the oven.
- Serve hot with a baguette, adding a little pesto to each mold.

Nutrition per serving: Calories: 249 Kcal | Fat: 21.6 g. | Protein: 9.6 g. | Carbs: 2.6 g.

14. Fried Eggs in Bread

Preparation Time: 10 minutes | serves: 1
Ingredients:
- 1 Egg
- 1 Bread, piece

Directions:
- From a slice of bread, cut the core and fry the resulting crust in a frying pan.
- Pour the egg in there and fry on both sides. Add tomatoes, ham, greens as desired.

Nutrition per serving: Calories: 200 Kcal | Fat: 6.7 g. | Protein: 10.2 g. | Carbs: 25.5 g.

15. Tomato-Basil Consommé

Preparation Time: 15 mins | Cooking Time: 5 mins | Number of Servings: 2

Ingredients:

- 2 tablespoons butter
- 1 cup diced onion
- 1 celery stalk, diced
- 1 carrot, chopped
- 2 garlic cloves, minced
- 1½ cups Vegetable Stock
- 1 (28-ounce) can whole tomatoes with their juices
- ¼ cup fresh basil
- 1 tablespoon tomato paste
- Pinch sugar
- ½ teaspoon kosher salt
- ¼ teaspoon freshly ground black pepper
- ⅓ cup shredded Parmesan cheese
- ½ cup heavy cream

Directions:

- Heat Up the pot and add butter. Add the onion, celery, and carrot and cook, stirring frequently, until softened, 3 to 4 minutes. Add the garlic and cook, stirring, until fragrant, 1 minute.
- Add the stock, tomatoes and their juices, basil, tomato paste, sugar, salt, and pepper. Stir to combine well.
- Leave to cook for 5 minutes, then add the Parmesan cheese and heavy cream and stir until fully combined and the cheese is melted. Season with salt and pepper. Serve with more cheese, crème fraîche, and crusty bread

Nutrition per serving: G Calories: 460 | Total fat: 33g | Saturated fat: 21g | Cholesterol: 102mg | Carbohydrates: 15g | Fiber: 4g | Protein: 21g

16. Banana Bread Smoothie

Number of servings: 1

Ingredients:

- 1 banana, sliced, frozen
- ¼ cup uncooked old-fashioned oats
- ½ teaspoon vanilla extract
- A pinch of ground nutmeg
- ½ cup almond milk
- ¼ cup plain, non-fat Greek yogurt
- ½ teaspoon pure maple syrup (optional)
- A pinch of ground cinnamon
- A bit of salt

Directions:

- Place banana, oats, vanilla, milk, yogurt, maple syrup, spices, and salt in a blender.
- Blend until you get a smooth puree.
- Pour into a glass and serve.

Nutrition per serving: Without maple syrup
Calories – 209 | Fat – 3 g | Carbohydrate – 24 g | Fiber – 5 g | Protein – 6 g

17. Oatmeal with Sun-Dried Tomato and Parmesan Cheese

Preparation time: 7 min / Cooking time: 8 min / Servings: 2

Ingredients:

- 1 cup, rolled oats
- 2 cups, vegetable or chicken stock
- 2 teaspoons, milled flaxseed
- 1 teaspoon, dried parsley
- 3 slices, sun-dried tomato
- 1/2 tablespoon, olive oil
- grated Parmesan cheese

Directions:

- Boil oatmeal and stock in a pot. Sprinkle in flaxseed. Cook for 8 minutes.
- Add in dried parsley to the cooked oatmeal.
- Finely chop sun-dried tomatoes.
- Serve oatmeal with olive oil, sun-dried tomato pieces, and grated Parmesan cheese.

Nutrition per serving: calories 180kcal | protein 2g | carbs 4g | fat 17g | fiber 2g

18. Crustless Tuna Breakfast Quiche

Preparation Time: 10 minutes | Cooking Time: 20 minutes | Serving: 6

Ingredients:

- 3 tablespoons oats
- ½ of a medium zucchini, grated
- 1 cup of canned tuna, drained
- ½ of a medium carrot, grated
- 1 tablespoon chopped basil
- ½ of a medium white onion, peeled, grated
- 1 tablespoon chopped dill
- ½ teaspoon salt
- 3 eggs
- ½ teaspoon ground black pepper

Directions:

- Switch on the oven, then set it to 350 degrees F and let it preheat.
- Take a medium bowl, crack the eggs in it, add remaining ingredients, and then stir until just mixed.
- Take a baking pan, line it with a parchment sheet, spoon the batter in it and then bake for 20 minutes until firm.
- Let the quiche cool completely, cut it into six slices, and then wrap each slice in plastic wrap and foil. Store in the refrigerator for up to 5 days or freeze for up to 1 month.
- When ready to eat, thaw a quiche slice overnight in the refrigerator, microwave for 2 to 3 and then serve.

Nutrition per Serving: Calories: 125 Cal | Total Fats: 6 g | Saturated Fat: 2 g | Carbohydrate: 4 g | Sugar: 1 g | Fiber: 1 g | Protein: 13 g

19. Apple Pancakes (Breakfast)

Number of servings: 6

Ingredients:

- 2 apples, peeled, cored, finely diced
- 2 cups oat milk
- 4 tablespoons maple syrup or honey
- ¼ teaspoon ground nutmeg
- 1 teaspoon baking powder
- 1 cup chopped mixed dried fruit and nuts
- 2 medium eggs
- 3 cups rolled oats or quick oats
- 4 teaspoons ground cinnamon

- ¼ teaspoon salt
- ¼ cup hemp seeds
- Olive oil cooking spray

Directions:

- Blend together oat milk, honey, nutmeg, baking powder, nuts, eggs, oats, cinnamon and salt in a blender until smooth.
- Pour into a bowl. Add hemp seeds and stir. Give the batter some rest for about 2-3 minutes.
- Place a nonstick pan over medium heat. When the pan is hot, spray the pan with cooking spray.
- Pour about ¼ cup of batter on the pan. Scatter a little of the apples over the batter (make 12 equal portions of the apple and scatter a portion of the apple).
- Press the apples lightly into the batter to adhere. Cook until the underside is golden brown.
- Turn the pancake over and cook the other side as well. Remove the pancake from the pan and keep warm.
- Make the remaining pancakes similarly (Steps 3-6, make sure to spray the pan each time you make a pancake). You should have 12 pancakes in all.
- Serve warm with a tablespoon of maple syrup for each serving, the nutritional value of which is not included.

Nutrition Per Serving: Two pancakes
Calories: 346 | Fat: 10 g | Carbohydrates: 54 g | Fiber: 8 g | Protein: 12 g

20. Chocolate Chip Oatmeal Cookie Smoothie

Number of servings: 1
Ingredients:

- 2/3 cup unsweetened almond milk
- ½ tablespoon chia seeds
- 2 medjool dates, pitted, soaked in warm water for 20 minutes
- 1 tablespoon raw cacao nibs or dark chocolate chips
- ¼ teaspoon pure vanilla extract
- Ice cubes, as required
- ¼ cup rolled oats
- ½ small banana, sliced, frozen
- 1 tablespoon almond butter
- ½ teaspoon cocoa powder, unsweetened
- 3-4 drops almond extract

Directions:

- Pour half the milk into a bowl. Add oats and chia seeds and stir. Chill for 2-8 hours.
- Pour the mixture into a blender. Add remaining milk, dates, cocoa powder, vanilla, banana, almond butter, cacao nibs, and almond extract and blend until smooth.
- Pour into a tall glass and serve

Nutrition per serving: Calories: 320 | Fat: 13.9 g | Carbohydrates: 44.8 g | Fiber: 7.7 g | Protein: 9.3 g

21. Sathu Mavu Recipe - Health Mix Powder for Adults Recipe

Preparation Time: 30 minutes | Cook Time: 5 minutes | Total Time: 35 minutes
Ingredients:

- Green Gram - 1/2 cup of

- Thinai / Foxtail Millet - 1/2 cup of
- Urad dal / Ulundu Paruppu - 1/4 cup of
- Horse Gram / Kollu - 1/2 cup of
- Rice - 1/4 cup of
- Roasted Gram Dal / Pottu kadalai - 1/2 cup of
- Wheat Flour - 1/2 cup of
- Ragi Flour - 1/2 cup of
- Yellow cornflour / Makkai ki Atta - 1/2 cup of
- Peanuts - 1/4 cup of
- Cashews - 1/4 cup of
- Badam / Almonds - 1/4 cup of
- Cardamom - 5 to 10
- Dry Ginger Powder - 2 tsp

FOR PORRIDGE:

- Health Mix powder - 3 tblsp
- Water or Milk - 1.5 cup of to 2 cups of
- Jaggery or Sugar to taste

Directions

- Except for gram dal, peanuts, almonds, cashews, and cardamom, dry roast all the grains. Dry roast till golden brown in a heavy bottom pan over low heat. Reduce the heat. Put it in a blender and finely powder it before transferring to a bowl.
- Now toast the gram dal, peanuts, cashews, badam, and cardamom in the same pan till brown, then cool. Put it in a blender and finely powder it before transferring it to the same bowl.
- Toss all of the flour into a bowl once it has been roasted till golden.
- Mix in the dried ginger powder well.
- This should be sieved and stored in a container.
- Take some powder, mix it with milk, and simmer until it thickens.
- Mix with the sweetener of your choosing.
- Serve the food.

22. Scrambled Eggs with Whole Grain Toast and Sliced Avocado

Preparation Time: 5 minutes | Cooking Time: 10 minutes | Servings: 2
Ingredients:

- 4 large eggs
- 2 slices of whole grain bread
- 1 ripe avocado, sliced
- 2 tablespoons of olive oil
- Salt and black pepper to taste

Directions:

- In a bowl, whisk together the eggs with a pinch of salt and black pepper.
- Heat a non-stick pan over medium heat and add 1 tablespoon of olive oil.
- Add the eggs to the pan and stir with a spatula until they start to set.
- Continue to stir the eggs until they are fully cooked and no longer runny.
- Toast the whole grain bread slices until they are lightly browned.
- Place the scrambled eggs on top of the toast slices.

- Top with sliced avocado and drizzle with the remaining olive oil.

Nutrition per serving: Calories: 365 | Total Fat: 25g | Saturated Fat: 5g | Cholesterol: 360mg | Sodium: 292mg | Carbohydrates: 18g | Fiber: 8g | Sugar: 2g | Protein: 19g

23. Cheesy Broccoli and Cauliflower Broth

Prep Time: 15 mins | Cooking Time: 8 mins | Number of Servings: 2
Ingredients:

- ½ tablespoon oil
- ½ large onion, chopped
- 1 cup chopped carrots
- 2 garlic cloves, minced
- 2 tablespoons flour
- 2 cups Vegetable Stock
- 2 cups chopped broccoli (including stems), plus 1 cup florets reserved
- 1 cup chopped cauliflower (including stems)
- 2 cups shredded low-fat Cheddar cheese
- ½ teaspoon paprika
- ¼ teaspoon nutmeg
- ½ cup whole milk
- Kosher salt
- Freshly ground black pepper

Directions:

- Preheat the pot then add the oil. Add the onion and carrots and cook until softened, 3 to 4 minutes. Add the garlic and flour and stir for 1 minute. Add the stock and continue stirring until no flour lumps remain.
- Add the 2 cups of chopped broccoli and the chopped cauliflower to the pot. Let it cook for 8 minutes.
- Using an immersion blender, carefully purée the soup until smooth. (Alternatively, you can use a countertop blender.)
- Then add the Cheddar cheese, paprika, and nutmeg and stir until fully combined and the cheese is melted. Stir in the milk and season with salt and pepper.
- Add the reserved 1 cup of broccoli florets and stir well, then loosely cover the pot and let sit for 4 to 5 minutes before serving.

Nutrition per Serving: Calories: 394 | Total fat: 14g | Saturated fat: 7g | Cholesterol: 30mg | Carbohydrates: 33g | Fiber: 6g | Protein: 35g

24. Omelet in Spanish

Preparation Time: 50 minutes | serves: 4
Ingredients:

- 1 lb. New Potato
- 6 Egg
- 5 fl. oz. Olive oil
- 1 Onion
- 3 tbsp. Parsley
- Pepper black ground, to taste

Directions:

- Peel new potatoes (you can leave the peel), cut into thick pieces. Finely chop the onion.
- Heat the oil in a pan, add the potatoes and onions, simmer over low heat, and cover with a lid, stirring for 30 minutes, until the potatoes are soft.
- Throw the potatoes and onions in a colander and save the drained oil. Separately, beat the eggs, then add the potatoes, parsley, and season with salt and pepper.
- Rest of the oil heat in a small saucepan. Transfer everything to a prepared frying pan and cook over low heat, leveling the omelet with a spatula.
- When the eggs grab, turn the omelet over on a plate, then let it slide into the pan and fry on the other side for a few minutes.
- Turn over again, fry on the other side, leveling with a spatula so that the omelet retains its shape. Transfer to a plate and chill for 10 minutes before serving.

Nutrition per serving: Calories: 207 Kcal Fat: 17.7 g. | Protein: 4.9 g. | Carbs: 7.2 g

25. Perfect Broccoli Scrambled Eggs

Prep Time: 2 minutes | Cook Time: 3 minutes | Total Time: 5 minutes
Ingredients:
For every serving:

- About 5 or 6 frozen broccoli florets
- 1 egg
- Red Robin Seasoning
- Freshly ground black pepper
- If desired: a small sprinkling of extra sharp cheddar cheese
- A tiny bit of butter

Direction:

- Cover the frozen broccoli with a plate in a shallow microwave-safe dish. Microwave for 1 minute on heavy. Stir it up a little. If it's already solidly frozen, microwave it for another 30 seconds to 1 minute, or until it's mostly thawed and wet in most areas.
- Remove the broccoli from the dish, leave the water in the bowl, then cut the broccoli into small pieces.
- In the bowl with the broccoli bath, crack the egg(s) and whisk until smooth. Season as need with salt and freshly ground black pepper.
- Rub a nonstick frying pan lightly with butter and cook over low heat. Pour the egg into the pan until it's warmed, then top with broccoli (and cheese, if you're using cheese). Let the egg to cook for a few minutes before it begins to set on the rim, then stir to loosen the egg from the pan's bottom.
- Pour the beautiful green scrambled eggs into a plate while the egg is just fried but still moist. If necessary, season with additional seasonings..

26. Mediterranean Pistachios and Fruits with Yogurt

Number of servings: 3
Ingredients:

- 6 tablespoons roasted, unsalted pistachios
- 1/8 cup chopped, dried apricots
- A pinch ground or grated nutmeg
- ½ teaspoon raw sugar
- 1 tablespoon dried pomegranate seeds or dried cranberries
- A pinch ground allspice
- 1/8 teaspoon cinnamon

- Greek yogurt to serve, as required

Directions:

- Place pistachios on a baking tray. Spread it evenly.
- Set up the temperature of your oven to 350° F and preheat the oven. Place the baking sheet in the oven and bake for about 7 minutes or until the nuts are toasted lightly.
- Cool the pistachios on your countertop.
- Transfer the pistachios into a bowl. Add pomegranate seeds, sugar, dried apricots, and all the spices. Toss well.
- Transfer into an airtight container. It can last for 6 – 7 days.
- To serve: Place yogurt in 3 serving bowls. 7. Add ¼ cup nut mixture in each bowl and serve.

Nutrition per serving: ¼ cup without yogurt
Calories – 116 | Fat – 7.1 g | Carbohydrate – 11 g | Fiber – 2.1 g | Protein – 3.5 g

27. Crispy Hash Breakfast Skillet

Prep Time: 40 minutes | Cook Time: 10 minutes | Total Time: 50 minutes
Ingredients:

- 2 medium Russet or Yukon Gold potatoes
- 3 strips bacon*
- 1 large bell pepper, chopped
- 1/4 tsp salt
- 1/4 tsp ground black pepper
- 4 large eggs*
- 1/3 cup of shredded smoked gouda cheese*
- optional: chopped fresh or dried parsley

Direction:

- Begin shredding the potatoes with your box grater's widest holes. Clean the potatoes by washing and scrubbing them. You can strip them or leave them on, depending on your preference. When I make shredded hash, I still peel them. In a big mixing bowl lined with paper towels, shred the potatoes. Add more paper towels on top and hold down firmly to retain as much moisture as possible. Continue squeezing and replacing paper towels as needed until much of the moisture is gone. You can also shred the potatoes, wrap them in a kitchen towel, and squeeze them out over the sink.
- Shred a potatoes and place them on a plate lined with two layers of paper towels. Cook for 2 minutes on high in the microwave (see notes in my post on why you're doing this). Remove the potatoes and set them aside.
- On the grill, heat a 10 – 12 inch skillet. Bacon can always be cooked in a cold skillet, so lay out your three strips on the pan before turning on the oven. Then reduce a heat to a low setting. Right until the bacon becomes crispy, cook it on both sides. They'll return to the stove before going into the oven, giving them more time to prepare later in this recipe. Remove a bacon from the heat and place it on a plate lined with paper towels to extract some of the grease. You should chop the bacon until it has cooled somewhat.
- Preheat the oven to 400 degrees Fahrenheit (204 degrees Celsius).

- Increase the heat on the stove to low. Attach the shredded potatoes until the bacon fat has started to boil. With the wooden spoon, stir them together quickly. Allow for about 2 minutes of cooking time, untouched. Mix the diced onion, salt, and pepper in a mixing bowl. Stir it around the couple of times, and use the back of a wooden spoon or spatula to flatten it out. Allow to cook for 3 minutes, uncovered. Enable to cook for another 2 minutes after stirring. At this stage, the potatoes should be well browned. If not, simmer for the few minutes longer, stirring occasionally, until they are. Cook for 2 minutes after adding the chopped bacon. Remove the skillet from the fire and use the back of a wooden spoon or spatula to flatten the surface of the hash. Create four shallow indentations in the hash with the back of a spoon. In every indentation, crack an egg. Serve with melted cheese on top (I usually sprinkle it around the eggs). Place the skillet in the oven and bake for 8-10 minutes, or until the egg whites have hardened. Season as needed with salt and pepper.

28. Quinoa Muffins

Preparation time: 10min / Cooking time: 30min / Servings: 12
Ingredients:

- 1 cup quinoa, rinsed
- 1/4 cup vegetable oil, such as safflower, plus more for pan
- 2 cups all-purpose flour, plus more for pan
- 3/4 cup packed dark-brown sugar
- 1 1/2 teaspoons baking powder
- 1 teaspoon salt
- 1/2 cup raisins
- 3/4 cup whole milk
- 1 large egg
- 1 teaspoon pure vanilla extract

Directions:

- Preheat oven to 350 degrees. In a medium saucepan, bring quinoa and 1 cup water to a boil. Reduce to a simmer; cover, and cook until water has been absorbed and quinoa is tender, 11 to 13 minutes.
- Meanwhile, brush a standard 12-cup muffin pan with oil; dust with flour, tapping out excess. In a medium bowl, whisk together flour, sugar, baking powder, salt, raisins, and 2 cups cooked quinoa; reserve any leftover quinoa for another use.
- In a small bowl, whisk together oil, milk, egg, and vanilla. Add milk mixture to flour mixture, and stir just until combined; divide batter among prepared muffin cups.
- Bake until toothpick inserted into the center of a muffin comes out clean, 25 to 30 minutes. Cool muffins in pan, 5 minutes; transfer to a wire rack to cool completely.

Nutrition per serving: calories 120kcal | protein 7g | carbs 10g | fat 5g | fiber 1g

29. Indian Masala Omelet Recipe

Cook Time: 20 mins
Ingredients:

- 4 eggs
- Kosher salt

- 1/2 tsp red chili powder
- 2 tbsp. chopped fresh cilantro leaves
- 2-3 small green chillis (such as Thai bird chilies) slit lengthwise
- 1 1/2 tbsp. finely chopped yellow onion
- 1 tbsp. finely chopped tomato
- 1 tbsp. vegetable oil, divided.

Directions

- With a sprinkle of flour, whisk the eggs. Chili powder, cilantro, chilies, onion, and tomato are added to the pot. 2 minutes of whisking until aerated and frothy
- In a heavy-bottomed nonstick 10-inch pan, cook 1/2 tbsp oil over medium heat until it shimmers. Gently pour in half of the omelette mixture and cook for 1 minute over medium heat. Flip gently and cook for another minute. Place on the plate and set aside to stay warm. Rep for the rest of the oil and egg combination. Serve right.

30. Oatmeal Banana Muffin

Preparation Time: 10 minutes | Cooking Time: 30 minutes | Serving: 4
Ingredients:
For the Muffins:

- 1 tablespoon flax meal
- 1 banana, peeled
- 1 cup oats
- 1 teaspoon baking soda
- 1 teaspoon vanilla extract, unsweetened
- 1 tablespoon honey
- 1/8 teaspoon salt
- 4 tablespoons almond butter
- 1 tablespoon yogurt
- 1 egg

For the Crumble:

- 4 ½ tablespoons oats
- 1/8 teaspoon salt
- 1 tablespoon honey
- 1 tablespoon almond butter

Directions:

- Switch on the oven, then set it to 350 degrees F and let it preheat.
- Meanwhile, take a medium bowl, place a banana in it, and mash it with a fork.
- Add honey, egg, yogurt, and butter, and then whisk until well combined.
- Add oats, flax meal, baking soda, and salt and stir until incorporated.
- Take six silicone muffin cups, line each cup with a muffin liner, and then fill them evenly with the prepared batter.
- Prepare the crumb mixture and for this, take a small bowl, place all of its ingredients in it, stir until mixed, and then sprinkle on top of the muffin batter.
- Place the prepared muffins into the oven and then bake for 25 to 30 minutes until firm and the top turn's golden brown.
- Meal Prep: Let the muffins cool completely, and then wrap each slice in plastic wrap and foil. Store each muffin

in the refrigerator for up to 5 days or freeze for up to 1 month.

- When ready to eat, thaw a muffin overnight in the refrigerator, microwave for 1 minute until warm, and then serve.

Nutrition per serving: Calories: 209 Cal | Total Fats: 11 g | Saturated Fat: 3 g | Carbohydrate: 24 g | Sugar: 9 g | Fiber: 3 g | Protein: 6 g

31. Cauliflower Tabbouleh with Chicken

Prep Time 10 Minutes | Cook Time 15 Minutes | Total Time 25 Minutes
Ingredients:

- Tabbouleh
- 1 medium head cauliflower
- 10.5 oz cherry tomatoes, quartered
- 1 medium cucumber, seeds removed then diced
- 1 cup of finely chopped parsley, tightly packed
- 1 tbsp The Fit Cook Land (OR dried oregano)
- 3 tbsp olive oil
- Juice from 1 lemon
- Sea salt & pepper to taste
- 4 tbsp crumbled feta (1 tbsp per serving, OPTIONAL)

Chicken:

- 1 1/4 lb chicken breast tenders
- 2 tsp The Fit Cook Everyday blend (OR 1 tsp garlic powder + 1 tsp onion powder)
- 2 tsp The Fit Cook Land (or Italian seasoning)
- 1 tbsp olive oil

Directions:

- In a large mixing bowl, grate the cauliflower head. Toss in the remaining tabbouleh ingredients and mix well. Season to taste with sea salts and pepper, then cover and refrigerate until ready to serve. It should be uniformly distributed among your meal containers, and fresh lemon should be garnished.
- Spices and mixes are used to season the chicken.
- Heat the nonstick skillet over medium-high heat, then add the oil.
- Cooks for 4 to 6 minutes on each side, or until the chicken is cooked through, before adding the chicken tenders.
- Divide the chicken into appropriate parts and combine with tabbouleh in the meal container. Add one tablespoon of feta cheese to each serving if preferred.
- Serve with a squeeze of fresh lemon as a garnish.

32. Banana, Raisin, and Walnut Baked Oatmeal

Number of servings: 3
Ingredients:

- 1 cup rolled oats
- ¾ teaspoon ground cinnamon
- ¼ teaspoon salt
- 1 cup low-fat milk
- 1 tablespoon canola oil
- ½ teaspoon vanilla extract
- 3 tablespoons raisins
- 3 tablespoons chopped walnuts

- ½ teaspoon baking powder
- 1/8 teaspoon ground allspice
- 6 tablespoons low-fat plain yogurt
- 2 tablespoons packed light brown sugar
- ½ large banana, cut into half-moon slices

Directions:
- You need to preheat your oven to 375°F. Grease a square baking dish of about (4-5 inches) with cooking spray.
- Add oats, baking powder, salt, walnuts, and allspice in a bowl and stir.
- Whisk together milk, oil, vanilla, yogurt, and brown sugar in another bowl. Once sugar dissolves, add raisins and banana slices and mix well.
- Transfer the liquid mixture into the bowl of oats and mix well. Spoon the mixture into the prepared baking dish.
- Place the baking dish in the oven and bake until golden brown on top. Cut into three equal portions and serve

Nutrition per serving: Calories: 327 | Fat: 13.1 g | Carbohydrates: 46.2 g | Fiber: 4.3 g | Protein: 9.1 g

33. Veggie Omelet with Bell Peppers, Onions, and Goat Cheese

Preparation Time: 5 minutes | Cooking Time: 15 minutes | Servings: 2

Ingredients:
- 4 big eggs
- 1/4 cup crumbled goat cheese
- 1/4 cup chopped red bell pepper
- 1/4 cup chopped green bell pepper
- 1/4 cup sliced yellow onion
- 1 tablespoonful extra-virgin olive oil
- 1/4 teaspoonful dried oregano
- Salt and black pepper to taste

Directions:
- In a small basin, beat the eggs with a fork until well mixed. Season with a pinch of salt and black pepper.
- Heat the olive oil in a non-stick skillet over medium heat. Add the bell peppers and onion and sauté for 2-3 minutes, until the vegetables are tender.
- Pour the beaten eggs into the skillet and let cook for about 1 minute, until the bottom is set. Sprinkle the goat cheese over the eggs, followed by the oregano.
- Use a spatula to gently fold the omelet in half, covering the cheese and vegetables. Cook for an additional 1-2 minutes, until the cheese is melted and the eggs are fully cooked.
- Cut the omelet in half and serve immediately.

Nutrition per serving: Calories: 280 | Protein: 18g | Carbohydrates: 8g | Fat: 20g | Fiber: 2g | Sodium: 340mg

CHAPTER 2: VEGETABLES AND SIDES

34. Pot Roast with Winter Root Vegetables

Ingredients:

- 2 tsp chopped fresh thyme
- 2 tsp Hungarian sweet paprika
- 2 tsp coarse kosher salt
- 2 tsp freshly ground black pepper
- 1 tsp dry mustard
- 1 tsp (packed) golden brown sugar
- 1 4-pound boneless grass-fed beef chuck roast, tied
- 6 ounces slab bacon, cut crosswise into 1/4-inch-thick slices, then into 1x1/2-inch rectangles
- 2 cups of dry red wine
- 1/2 cup of low-salt chicken broth
- 2 large onions, thinly sliced
- 12 small shallots, peeled
- 12 garlic cloves, peeled
- 3 bay leaves
- 4 large carrots (about 1 pound), peeled, cut into 1-inch pieces
- 3 medium parsnips (about 12 ounces), peeled, cut into 1-inch pieces
- 1 small celery root, peeled, cut into 1-inch cubes

Direction:

- Preheat the oven to 350 degrees Fahrenheit. In a shallow mixing bowl and combine the first six ingredients. Rub the spice mixture all over the meat.
- In a heavy large ovenproof kettle, cook bacon until browned and finely crisped over medium heat. Switch the bacon to paper towels to rinse using a slotted spoon. Remove all but 2 tablespoons of drippings from the pot. Raise the temperature to medium-high. Cook until the beef is browned on both sides, about 12 minutes. Place the beef on a tray. Bring red wine to a boils in the pot, brushing off any browned parts. Boil for 5 minutes and or until the liquid has been reduced to 1/2 cup. Add the broth and bacon to the pot. Place the beef on tops of the bacon. Surround the beef with carrots, shallots, garlic, and bay leaves.
- Cover the kettle, place it in the oven, and roast for 1 hour. Turn the beef over and whisk in the onions. Cover and continue to roast for another hour, adding 1/4 cup of water if necessary. Place the beef on a tray. Stir in the onions, parsnips, and celery to coat. Place the beef on tops of the vegetables, cover, and roast for another 45 minutes or until the beef and vegetables are tender. Place the beef on a serving platter. Remove the fat from the sauce's crust. Season sauce with salt, pepper as needed. Serve the beef with the gravy.

35. Eggplant in Sesame

Preparation time: 15 minutes | serves: 4

Ingredients:

- 2 Eggplant
- 5 tbsp Sesame seeds
- 1 Egg
- 2 tbsp Olive oil

Directions:

- Eggplant cut into slices half a centimeter thick and salt.
- Beat the egg, soak the eggplant in it and roll in the sesame.
- Fry in oil on both sides until golden brown, and then spread on a napkin so that excess oil is absorbed.
- Serve hot.

Nutrition per serving: Calories: 187 Kcal | Fat: 16 g. | Protein: 5.2 g. | Carbs: 6.9 g.

36. Ravioli & Vegetable Soup

Number of servings: 2

Ingredients:

- ½ tablespoon extra-virgin olive oil
- 1 clove garlic, minced
- ½ can (from 28 ounces can) crushed tomatoes, fire roasted ones if possible
- ¾ cup hot water
- ½ package (from an 8 – 9 ounces package) fresh or frozen cheese and whole wheat ravioli
- Freshly ground pepper to taste
- 1 cup frozen bell pepper and onion mix, thawed, diced
- Crushed red pepper to taste
- 1 cup vegetable or chicken broth
- ½ teaspoon dried basil or marjoram
- 1 medium
- 1 medium zucchini, diced
- Salt to taste

Directions:

- Place a soup pot over medium flame. Pour oil into the pot and let it heat. When the oil is heated, add the onion-pepper mixture, crushed red pepper, and garlic and stir-fry for about a minute.
- Stir in basil, tomatoes, and broth and raise the heat to high heat. When the mixture begins to boil, add ravioli and cook for about 3 minutes less than that mentioned on the package.
- Stir in zucchini and cook for a couple of minutes until zucchini is slightly tender. Add salt and pepper to taste. 4. Ladle into soup bowls and serve

Nutrition per serving: 2 cups

Calories – 261 | Fat – 8.3 g | Carbohydrate – 32.6 g | Fiber – 7 g | Protein – 10.6 g

37. Cacio e Pepe Spaghetti Squash

Prep Time: 15 mins | Cooking Time: 7 mins | Number of Servings: 2

Ingredients:

- 1 whole spaghetti squash
- Kosher salt
- 3 tablespoons unsalted butter
- 1 teaspoon freshly squeezed lemon juice
- ½ cup Pecorino Romano cheese
- ¼ cup Parmesan cheese, plus more for serving
- 1½ teaspoons freshly ground black pepper

Directions:

- Using a hefty, sharp knife, carefully cut the spaghetti squash in half lengthwise (this will result in long strands of squash flesh). With a spoon, scrape out the seeds in the middle.

- Place a trivet or steamer basket in the pressure cooker pot; add 1 cup of water and half of the squash. (Wrap the other half in plastic wrap and refrigerate for another meal.)
- Secure the lid and cook on high pressure for 7 minutes, using a quick release at the end of the cooking time. Select cancel and open the lid carefully.
- Transfer the spaghetti squash to a work surface and let cool until it can be handled. Using a fork or large spoon, gently pull the flesh away from the skin and break into long spaghetti-like strands.
- Remove the trivet from the cooker pot. Select sauté and adjust to low. Season the water with salt. Add the butter and lemon juice and stir until melted.
- Gradually sprinkle in the Pecorino Romano cheese and stir until completely melted. Repeat with the ¼ cup of Parmesan cheese. Add the spaghetti squash strands and stir until the cheese is melted and smooth (the cheese will initially clump before melting into a sauce). Stir in the pepper and season with salt. Serve topped with more Parmesan cheese.

Nutrition per serving: Calories: 509 | Total fat: 40g | Saturated fat: 29g | Cholesterol: 126mg | Carbohydrates: 12g | Fiber: 3g | Protein: 24g

38. Spicy Cauliflower Rice with Ground Turkey

Preparation Time: 5 minutes | Cooking Time: 15 minutes | Serving: 2

Ingredients:
- 6 ounces ground turkey
- 2 teaspoons paprika
- 3 cups cauliflower rice
- ½ teaspoon ground black pepper
- 1 medium carrot, peeled, chopped
- 1 teaspoon crushed red pepper flakes
- Salt as needed
- ½ of a medium red bell pepper, cored, chopped
- 2 teaspoons minced garlic
- ½ teaspoon turmeric
- 1 teaspoon ground cumin
- 1 tablespoon pickled Jalapeno
- 1/3 cup water
- ½ teaspoon ground coriander
- 2 tablespoons olive oil

Directions
- Take a large skillet pan, place it over medium-high heat, pour in water, add turkey and then cook for 5 minutes until thoroughly cooked.
- Add ½ teaspoon minced garlic along with turmeric, black pepper, red pepper flakes, cumin, coriander, and 1 teaspoon paprika and then cook for 3 minutes or until cooking liquid has been evaporated.
- Switch heat to medium level, add bell pepper, carrot, cauliflower rice, 1 teaspoon salt, and 1 tablespoon oil, stir until mixed, and then cook for 4 minutes, covering the pan with its lid.
- Then stir in remaining garlic and oil, along with jalapeno, and continue cooking for 2 minutes.

- Meal Prep: Let the cauliflower rice with turkey cool completely, then divide them evenly between two meal prep containers and cover it with a lid.
- Store the containers in the refrigerator for up to 5 days or freeze for up to 1 month.
- When ready to eat, thaw the container overnight in the refrigerator, microwave for 2 to 3 minutes until hot, and then serve.

Nutrition per Serving: Calories: 443 Cal | Total Fats: 31 g | Saturated Fat: 6 g | Carbohydrate: 18 g | Sugar: 6 g | Fiber: 7 g | Protein: 28 g

39. Quinoa with Eggs and Vegetables

Preparation time: 10min / Cooking time: 15min / Servings: 2

Ingredients:
- 1 medium bell pepper red, yellow, or orange
- 1 medium carrot
- 1 jalapeno pepper
- 1 tbsp grapeseed oil or other kind
- 2 tbsp soy sauce
- 3 eggs
- 2 cups cooked quinoa
- ¼ cup chopped scallion

Directions:
- Prep the vegetables. Cut the peppers into strips. Using a vegetable peeler, shave the carrot into flat strips. Then, dice the jalapeño pepper.
- Place a non-stick skillet over medium-high heat and add the oil and bell pepper. Cook for 3 minutes, until the pepper just starts to soften.
- Add the carrot strips and jalapeño, and then cook for another 2 minutes.
- Add the soy sauce and eggs to the pan and cook until the eggs are almost set. At this point, add the cooked quinoa and cook until heated through.
- Stir in the scallions and serve immediately. Garnish with sliced jalapeno, if desired.

Nutrition per serving: calories 422kcal | protein 19g | carbs 48g | fat 17g | fiber 8g

40. Swift Fried Rice

Prep Time: 20 mins | Cooking Time: 15 mins | Number of Servings: 2

Ingredients:
- ½ cup jasmine rice rinsed well
- ¾ cup of water
- ½ tablespoon oil
- ¼ cup diced yellow onion
- ½ tablespoon unsalted butter
- ¼ cup chopped carrots
- ¼ cup green peas
- 1 egg, lightly beaten
- 1 tablespoon low-sodium soy sauce
- 1 scallion, chopped
- Sesame seeds, for garnish

Directions:
- Add the rice and water to the pot and Stir.

- Secure the lid and cook on high pressure for 12 minutes, then allowing the pressure to release naturally, 10 minutes. Carefully remove the lid. Press cancel.
- Fluff the rice with a fork and transfer to a medium bowl; cover and set aside.
- Add the oil to the pot and heat until the display reads hot, and then add the onion. Cook for 2 minutes, stirring frequently until softened. Add the butter, carrots, and peas and cook for 2 minutes.
- Move the veggies to the side of the pot and pour the beaten egg into the empty side. Stir constantly as the egg scrambles to avoid sticking. Once the egg is almost cooked, stir it into the vegetables.
- Stir in the cooked rice, soy sauce, and scallion. Cook everything together for 8 to 10 minutes, stirring occasionally. Portion into bowls and sprinkle with sesame seeds.

Nutrition per serving:
Calories: 299 | Total fat: 9g | Saturated fat: 3g | Cholesterol: 86mg | Carbohydrates: 45g | Fiber: 3g | Protein: 8g

41. Pasta with Asparagus

Preparation Total Time: 20 min | makes: 6 servings
Ingredients:
- 5 garlic cloves, minced
- ¼ to ½ tsp crushed red pepper flakes
- 2 to 3 dashes hot pepper sauce
- ¼ cup of olive oil
- 1 tbsp butter
- 1 pound asparagus, cutted into 1-1/2-inch pieces
- Salt as need
- ¼ tsp pepper
- ¼ cup of shredded Parmesan cheese
- ½ pound mostaccioli, cooked and drained

Directions:
- In a large cast-iron or other strong skillet, cook garlic, red pepper flakes and hot pepper sauce for 1 minute. Add the asparagus, salt and pepper; cook until crisp-tender, 8-10 mins. Add cheese. Add hot pasta and toss to cover. Serve instantly.

Nutrition info 1 cup of: 259 calories | 13g fat | 8mg cholesterol | 83mg sodium | 30g carbohydrate | 7g protein

42. Vegetable Frittata

Preparation Time: 10 minutes | Cooking Time: 20 minutes | Serving: 8
Ingredients:
- 1 small red bell pepper, cored, chopped
- ½ teaspoon salt 1 small zucchini, ends trimmed, small diced
- ¼ teaspoon ground black pepper 2 green onions, chopped
- ¼ teaspoon baking powder 4 ounces broccoli, cut into small florets
- ⅓ cup feta cheese, crumbled 7 eggs
- ⅓ cup chopped parsley
- 3 tablespoons olive oil and more as needed
- 1 teaspoon thyme
- ¼ cup almond milk, unsweetened

Directions:
- Switch on the oven, place a rimmed baking sheet in it, then set the temperature to 450 degrees F and let it preheat.
- Take a large bowl, place broccoli, bell pepper, zucchini, onion, salt, black pepper, and oil, and then stir until well coated.
- Remove the hot rimmed baking sheet from the oven, spread the vegetable mixture on it in an even layer, return the baking sheet into the oven and cook for 15 minutes.
- Meanwhile, take another bowl, crack eggs in it, add baking powder, thyme, feta cheese, parsley, some salt, and black pepper, pour in the milk and then whisk until combined.
- After 15 minutes, transfer vegetables to the egg bowl and then switch heat to 400 degrees F.
- Take an oven-proof skillet pan, coat it with oil, place the pan over medium heat and when hot, pour the egg-vegetable mixture in it and then cook for 3 minutes until eggs begin to settle.
- Then transfer the pan into the oven and bake for 10 minutes until firm and top turn golden.
- Meal Prep: Let the frittata cool completely, cut it into eight slices, and then wrap each slice in plastic wrap and foil.
- Store each frittata slice in the refrigerator for up to 5 days or freeze for up to 1 month.
- When ready to eat, thaw a frittata slice overnight in the refrigerator, microwave for 2 to 3 minutes until hot, and then serve.

Nutrition per serving: Calories: 136.3 Cal | Total Fats: 10.2 g | Saturated Fat: 2.6 g | Carbohydrate: 4.2 g | Sugar: 1.3 g | Fiber: 1.1 g | Protein: 7.8 g

43. Easy Sautéed Kale

Preparation time: 5 mins | Cook Time: 5 mins | Total Time: 10 mins | serves: 6
Ingredients:
- 10-ounce bag of chopped kale (roughly 5 cups of)
- ¼ cup of water
- 2 Tbsp. nutritional yeast
- 2 tsp. garlic powder
- Juice of half a lemon
- Salt as need (optional)

Directions:
- Turn on a nonstick skillet.
- Add the kale to the pan, then add the water to cook it. Cooking the kale until it turns light orange. You can cook the kale in batches if you don't have a big enough skillet. Divide the water for each batch similarly.
- Cook the kale, tossing it with the nutritional yeast and garlic powder. Drizzle with lemon juice and eat.
- Try these toppings on your kale: Organic Parmesan, Garlic Lemon Tahini Sauce, Lemon Wedges, and Red Pepper Flakes.

Nutrition info Serves 6 Calories per Serving: 19 Total | Fat 0.2g | Cholesterol 0mg | Sodium 8mg | Total Carbohydrate 3.7g | Dietary Fiber 0.9g | Sugars 0.8g | Protein 1.5g | Vitamin C 23.9mg | Calcium 22mg | Iron 0.3mg

44. Veggie Omelet

Number of servings: 2
Ingredients:

- 1 tablespoon extra-virgin olive oil
- 1 clove garlic, minced
- ½ small onion, thinly sliced
- ½ cup shredded cabbage
- 4.5 ounces diced, diced, mixed, cooked vegetables of your preference or leftover cooked vegetables
- 3 large eggs
- ½ tablespoon finely chopped flat-leaf parsley
- Salt to taste
- 2 ounces soft goat cheese
- Pepper to taste

Directions:

- Add oil into a pan and heat over medium flame. Add onion and cook until pink. Stir in garlic and cook for a few seconds.
- Stir in cabbage and cooked vegetables. Stir-fry for a couple of minutes.
- Beat eggs with salt and pepper. Pour into the skillet, all over the vegetables. Add parsley and stir lightly. Now do not stir anymore.
- Cook until the edges are set and the underside is golden brown. Carefully lift the omelet with a spatula and turn the omelet over.
- Sprinkle cheese on top. Cook for a couple of minutes.
- Cut into 2 halves and serve

Nutrition per serving: Calories – 259 | Fat – 13 g | Carbohydrate – 22 g | Fiber – 3 g | Protein – 15 g

45. Balsamic Roasted Carrots and Baby Onions

Preparation time: 10 mins | Cook: 50 mins | Servings: 8
Ingredients

- 2 bunches baby (Dutch) carrots, scrubbed, ends trimmed to 3cm
- 16 small (60g each) white onions, peeled, halved
- 1 tbsp. extra virgin olive oil
- 45g (1/4 cup of, lightly packed) brown sugar
- 2 tbsp. balsamic vinegar

Direction:

- Heat the oven to 190°C. Cover a baking sheet with non-stick material.
- Place the vegetables, onion and oil in a big bowl and blend well. Arrange the carrots and onions in a single layer. Bake for 20 mins or until tender.
- Sprinkle a combination of sugar and vinegar over it. Roast at this temperature for about 30 mins. Season with salt and pepper.

46. Mushroom Risotto

Prep Time: 20 mins | Cooking Time: 5 mins | Number of Servings: 2
Ingredients:

- 1 tablespoon oil
- 8 ounces cremini mushrooms, sliced
- ¼ teaspoon kosher salt
- 2 shallots, chopped
- 2 garlic cloves, minced
- 1 cup Arborio rice
- ½ cups dry white wine, such as Chardonnay or Chablis
- 3 cups Vegetable Stock
- ½ teaspoon fresh thyme
- 2 tablespoons unsalted butter
- 2 cups fresh baby spinach (optional)
- ¼ cup freshly grated Parmesan cheese, plus more for garnish

Directions

- Select the sauté setting on the pressure cooker. Heat the oil in the cooker pot until the display reads hot. Add the mushrooms and salt and cook for 8 minutes, or until the mushrooms are tender, stirring frequently.
- Add the shallots and garlic and cook for 3 minutes more, stirring often.
- Add the rice and cook for 3 to 4 minutes, stirring often, until the rice kernel edges start to become translucent.
- Add the wine and cook, stirring, until the alcohol aroma has cooked off and the wine has almost fully evaporated about 2 minutes.
- Add the stock and thyme. Make sure all of the ingredients are submerged.
- Secure the lid and cook on low pressure for 5 minutes, using a quick release at the end of the cooking time. Carefully remove the lid.
- Add the butter and spinach (if using) to the rice mixture and stir to wilt the spinach. Stir in the ¼ cup of Parmesan cheese and season with salt if desired. Serve with an additional sprinkle of cheese.

Nutrition per Serving: Calories: 702 | Total fat: 24g | Saturated fat: 12g | Cholesterol: 49mg | Carbohydrates: 85g | Fiber: 3g | Protein: 22g

47. Baked Cod and Veggies

Preparation Time: 10 minutes | Cooking Time: 25 minutes | Serving: 4
Ingredients:

- 1-pound Atlantic cod, cleaned, divided into 4 pieces
- 1 teaspoon salt
- 2 cups cherry tomatoes
- 1 teaspoon ground black pepper
- 2 cups purple potatoes, diced
- 4 tablespoons olive oil
- 1 teaspoon Italian seasoning mix

Directions:

- Switch on the oven, then set it to 400 degrees F and let it preheat. Meanwhile, take a medium bowl, place potatoes in it, add 2 tablespoons oil and then toss until coated.
- Take a baking sheet, scatter potatoes on it in a single layer and then bake for 15 minutes until roasted. When done, push the potatoes to one side of the sheet and place the cod pieces and cherry tomato on the other side of the sheet.
- Drizzle remaining oil over cod pieces and tomatoes, and then season potatoes, tomatoes, and cod with salt, black pepper, and Italian seasoning mix. Return the baking

sheet into the oven and then continue baking for 12 minutes until thoroughly cooked.

- Meal Prep: Let the cod and vegetables cool completely, then divide it evenly among four meal prep containers and cover it with a lid. Store the containers in the refrigerator for up to 5 days or freeze for up to 1 month.
- When ready to eat, thaw the container overnight in the refrigerator, microwave for 2 to 3 minutes until hot, and then serve.

Nutrition per Serving: Calories: 267 Cal | Total Fats: 11 g | Saturated Fat: 3 g | Carbohydrate: 19 g | Sugar: 3 g | Fiber: 5 g | Protein: 23 g

48. Broccoli-Cheddar Scalloped Potatoes

Prep Time: 20 mins | Cooking Time: 5 mins | Number of Servings: 2
Ingredients:

- 1½ tablespoons unsalted butter, divided
- ¼ yellow onion, chopped
- ¾ cup Chicken Stock
- ½ teaspoon garlic powder
- ¼ teaspoon kosher salt
- Pinch freshly ground black pepper
- 3 medium Yukon Gold potatoes, sliced ⅛ inch thick
- 1 cup broccoli florets, chopped
- 3 tablespoons sour cream
- ½ cup shredded Cheddar cheese, divided
- ⅓ cup shredded Monterey Jack cheese, divided

Directions:

- Melt 1 tablespoon of butter in the pot until hot. Add the onion and cook for 4 to 5 minutes, or until softened, then stir in the stock, garlic powder, salt, and pepper.
- Place a steamer basket in the pot. Add the potatoes and broccoli. Secure the lid and cook on high pressure for 5 minutes, using a quick release at the end of the cooking time. Select cancel and open the lid. Carefully remove the steamer basket from the pot.
- Preheat the oven broiler. Coat a small ovenproof casserole dish with the remaining ½ tablespoon of butter. Transfer the potatoes and broccoli to the prepared dish.
- To the cooking liquid in the cooker pot, add the sour cream, half of the Cheddar cheese, and half of the Monterey Jack cheese and stir until melted and smooth. Pour over the potatoes and broccoli, making sure not to come above the top edge of the dish.
- Top with the remaining cheeses, place in a baking pan and broil until golden brown, 6 to 7 minutes.

Nutrition per Serving: Calories: 325| Total fat: 22g| Saturated fat: 14g| Cholesterol: 62mg| Carbohydrates: 18g| Fiber: 4g| Protein: 15g

49. Mediterranean Chicken Thighs

Preparation Time: 10 minutes | Cooking Time: 55 minutes | Serving: 4

Ingredients:

- 1 ½ pounds potatoes, scrubbed, cut into small chunks
- 8 chicken thighs
- 4 teaspoons minced garlic
- ¾ teaspoon salt
- ¼ cup capers, drained
- ½ teaspoon ground black pepper
- 4 tablespoons olive oil
- 1 pint of cherry tomatoes
- 1 teaspoon dried oregano
- 10 ounces roasted red peppers, drained, sliced
- 3 tablespoons chopped parsley

Directions

- Switch on the oven, then set it to 400 degrees F and let it preheat. Meanwhile, wash the chicken thighs, pat dry, and then season with salt and black pepper
- Take a skillet pan, place it over medium-high heat, add oil, and when hot, add the seasoned chicken thigh pieces and then cook for 4 to 5 minutes per side until golden.
- Meanwhile, take a large bowl, place potatoes in it, add capers, red pepper, garlic, tomatoes, oregano, some more salt, black pepper, and oil, and then toss until mixed.
- Take a baking sheet, spread the potatoes mixture on it in an even layer, and then bake for 45 to 55 minutes until cooked, tossing halfway.
- Meal Prep: Let the chicken thighs and roasted potato mixture cool completely, then divide them evenly among four meal prep containers and cover it with a lid.
- Store the containers in the refrigerator for up to 5 days or freeze for up to 1 month.
- When ready to eat, thaw the container overnight in the refrigerator, microwave for 2 to 3 minutes until hot, and then serve.

Nutrition per Serving: Calories: 647 Cal | Total Fats: 38 g | Saturated Fat: 10 g | Carbohydrate: 34 g | Sugar: 3 g | Fiber: 8 g | Protein: 44 g

50. One Pan Honey Garlic Chicken and Veggies

Preparation Time: 10 Minutes | Cook Time: 35 Minutes | Total Time: 45 Minutes

Ingredients:

- 3 tbsp. olive oil, divided
- 2 tbsp. unsalted butter, melted
- 2 tbsp. honey
- 2 tbsp. brown sugar
- 1 tbsp. Dijon mustard
- 3 cloves garlic, minced
- 1/2 tsp dried oregano
- 1/2 tsp dried basil Kosher salt, freshly ground black pepper, as need
- 16 ounces baby red potatoes, halved
- 4 boneless, skinless chicken breasts
- 24 ounces broccoli florets*
- 2 tbsps. chopped fresh parsley leave

Directions:

- Preheat the oven to 400 degrees Fahrenheit. Cover a baking sheet with nonstick spray or lightly oil it.
- 2 tbsps. olive oil, butter, honey, brown sugar, Dijon, garlic, oregano, and basil in a small bowl; season with salt and pepper as required. Remove from the equation.
- Place the potatoes in a singles layer on the baking sheet that has been prepared. Season with salt, pepper as needed and drizzle with the remaining 1 tbsp olive oil. Brush each chicken breast with the honey mixture and arrange in a single sheet.
- Place the chicken in the oven and roast for around 25-30 minutes and until it reaches an internal temperatures of 165 F. During the last 10 minutes of preparation, add the broccoli. Then broil for 2- 3 minutes, or until mildly charred and caramelized.
- If needed, garnish with parsley before serving.

51. Herb and Lemon Roasted Chicken

Preparation time: 30min / Cooking time: 1h/ Servings: 4

Ingredients:

- 2 tablespoons unsalted butter, softened
- 5 garlic cloves, 1 minced
- 1/2 teaspoon minced rosemary plus 2 rosemary sprigs
- 1/2 teaspoon minced thyme plus 2 thyme sprigs
- 1/2 teaspoon finely grated lemon zest
- Salt and freshly ground pepper
- One 4-pound chicken, at room temperature
- 1 large onion, cut into 8 wedges
- 1 lemon, cut crosswise into 8 rounds
- 1/2 cup chicken stock or low-sodium broth

Directions:

- Preheat the oven to 425° and position a rack in the lower third of the oven. In a bowl, mix the butter with the minced garlic, minced herbs and the lemon zest and season with salt and pepper.
- Pat the chicken dry. Rub half of the herb butter under the skin and the rest over the chicken; season with salt and pepper.
- Set the chicken breast-side-up on a rack in a roasting pan. Scatter the onion, lemon, garlic cloves and herb sprigs and add 1/2 cup of water. Roast for 30 minutes, until the breast is firm and just beginning to brown in spots. Using tongs, turn the chicken breast-down and roast for 20 minutes longer, until the skin is lightly browned.
- Using tongs, turn the chicken breast-side-up. Add another 1/2 cup of water. Roast for about 20 minutes longer, until an instant-read thermometer inserted in the inner thigh registers 175° to 180°.
- Tilt the chicken to drain the cavity juices into the pan; transfer the bird to a cutting board. Remove the rack from the pan and spoon off the fat. Set the pan over high heat. Add the stock and cook, scraping up any browned bits. Press the lemon to release the juices. Carve the chicken and pass the chunky jus at the table.

Nutrition per serving: calories 510kcal | protein 71g | carbs 4g | fat 31g

52. Lemon Chicken Skewers

Preparation Time: 10 minutes | Cooking Time: 10 minutes | Serving: 6

Ingredients:

- 1 1/2 pounds chicken breasts, boneless, skinless, 1-inch cubed
- 3/4 teaspoon salt
- 2 teaspoons dried oregano
- 3 tablespoons lemon juice
- 1/8 teaspoon ground black pepper
- 1 tablespoon red wine vinegar
- 1/2 teaspoon ground coriander
- 1 tablespoon olive oil
- 1/2 teaspoon dried parsley
- 1 teaspoon minced garlic

Directions:

- Take a large bowl, place chicken pieces in it, add the remaining ingredients, and then stir until coated.
- Cover the bowl with its lid, place it in the refrigerator and let it rest for a minimum of 45 minutes.
- When ready to cook, take a griddle pan, place it over medium-high heat, grease it with oil and let it preheat.
- Thread the marinated chicken pieces on skewers, place them on the griddle pan and then cook for 4 to 5 minutes per side until thoroughly cooked and developed grill marks.
- Meal Prep: Let the chicken skewers cool completely, then divide them evenly among six meal prep containers and cover them with a lid.
- Store the container in the refrigerator for up to 5 days or freeze for up to 1 month. When ready to eat, thaw the container overnight in the refrigerator, microwave for 2 to 3 minutes until hot, and then serve.

Nutrition per serving: Calories: 268 Cal | Total Fats: 7 g | Saturated Fat: 2 g | Carbohydrate: 11 g | Sugar: 7 g | Fiber: 1 g | Protein: 40 g

53. Spicy Brown Mustard Chicken

Preparation time: 15 mins | Total Cook Time: 1 hr. 15 mins Servings: 4

Ingredients

- 4 skinless, boneless chicken breast halves
- ½ cup of spicy brown mustard
- ½ cup of Italian seasoned bread crumbs
- ¼ cup of butter, melted
- 2 tbsps. lemon juice
- 2 tbsps. water
- Paprika as need

Directions

- Heat oven to 350F. Heat a baking bowl.
- Brush the chicken on every sides with the mustard. Place bread crumbs in bowl. Press the chicken onto the bread crumbs uniformly. Arrange the chicken in the cooked oven.
- In a bowl, mix the sugar, lemon juice, and water. Roll each chicken breast in the marinade mixture. Pour the excess mixture over the breasts.

- Bake at 450 degrees for 45 mins. Turn on, stir, and bake for 15 mins.

Nutrition per Serving: 324 calories| protein 28.8g| carbohydrates 13.5g| fat 17.2g| cholesterol 97.9mg| sodium 793.8mg.

54. Chicken with Tomatoes, Prunes, Cinnamon, and Wine

Preparation time: 70 minutes | serves: 6

Ingredients:

- 1 Chicken
- 9 oz Tomatoes
- 9 fl. oz Dry white wine
- 16 Prunes without stones
- 5 fl. oz Water
- 2.5 tbsp Butter
- 2 tbsp Red wine vinegar
- 2 tsp Sugar
- 1 Cinnamon, stick

Directions:

- Cut the carcass of the chicken into 8 parts, salt, and pepper to taste. Fry the pieces in butter in a heavy skillet for 5 minutes. After roasting, put all the chicken pieces tightly in the pan, add the wine and bring to a boil.
- Boil for 4 minutes until the liquid has evaporated to about half. Add water to the pan, add peeled and chopped tomatoes, 1 cinnamon stick, 3/4 teaspoon salt, 1/4 teaspoon pepper and bring to a boil again. Continue to cook, covered with a lid, on low heat for 20 minutes.
- Add the chopped prunes, vinegar and sugar, and bring to the boil again. After turning down the heat, cover and cook for 10 minutes. Remove the pieces of chicken from the pan, put on a dish and cover with foil. Bring the sauce remaining in the pan to a boil and cook on high heat for 8-10 minutes.
- The sauce should thicken and evaporate to about 300 ml. Lay the chicken on plates at the rate of 2 pieces per 1 person.
- Serve with cooked tomato and prune sauce.

Nutrition per serving: Calories: 160 Kcal | Fat: 9.5 g. | Protein: 11.3 g. | Carbs: 5.8 g.

55. Chicken & Carrot Soup

Preparation time: 10min / Cooking time: 15min / Servings: 4

Ingredients:

- 1 tbsp. – oil
- 1 - onion, chopped finely
- 2 - carrots, sliced
- 3 - stalks celery, cut into small size
- Salt as per taste
- Pepper as per taste
- 5 - cups chicken stock
- 2 - boneless chicken breast halves

Directions:

- Heat oil. Fry onion till transparent.
- Add chicken stock and bring to a boil.
- Add carrots, celery, chicken breast, and salt.

- Let it cook till the vegetables and chicken are tender (approximately -10 minutes).
- Remove from fire. Remove the chicken breast, and let it cool.
- Cut into bite-sized pieces. Add back to stock.
- Add pepper and bring back to a boil.

Nutrition per serving: calories 240kcal | fat 9g

56. Chicken & Carrot Soup

Preparation time: 10min / Cooking time: 15min / Servings: 4
Ingredients:

- 1 tbsp. – oil
- 1 - onion, chopped finely
- 2 - carrots, sliced
- 3 - stalks celery, cut into small size
- Salt as per taste
- Pepper as per taste
- 5 - cups chicken stock
- 2 - boneless chicken breast halves

Directions:

- Heat oil. Fry onion till transparent.
- Add chicken stock and bring to a boil.
- Add carrots, celery, chicken breast, and salt.
- Let it cook till the vegetables and chicken are tender (approximately -10 minutes).
- Remove from fire. Remove the chicken breast, and let it cool.
- Cut into bite-sized pieces. Add back to stock.
- Add pepper and bring back to a boil.

Nutrition per serving: calories 240kcal | fat 9g

57. Skillet Lemon Chicken & Potatoes with Kale

Number of servings: 8
Ingredients:

- 6 tablespoons extra-virgin olive oil, divided
- 1 teaspoon salt, divided
- 2 pounds baby Yukon gold potatoes, halved lengthwise
- 2 large lemons, cut lemons, cut into thin, round slices, deseeded
- 2 tablespoons chopped fresh tarragon
- 2 pound boneless, skinless, chicken thighs, trimmed
- 1 teaspoon pepper, divided
- 1 cup low sodium chicken broth
- 8 cloves garlic, minced
- 12 cups baby kale

Directions:

- Set up the temperature of your oven to 400° F and preheat the oven.
- Place a large, cast-iron skillet over medium-high flame. Add 2 tablespoons of oil and let it heat.
- Sprinkle ½ teaspoon salt and ½ teaspoon pepper all over the chicken and place in the pan.
- Cook until brown all over. Remove chicken from the pan and place it on a plate.
- Pour 4 tablespoons of oil into the skillet and let it heat. Add potatoes, ½ teaspoon salt, and ½ teaspoon pepper

and mix well. Now cook the potatoes until brown, on the cut part of the potato pieces.

- Add broth, garlic, lemon slices, and tarragon and mix well. Add the chicken into the skillet. Turn off the heat.
- Mix well and shift the skillet into the oven. Bake until the potatoes are fork-tender and the chicken is well-cooked inside.
- Add kale and stir. Bake for about 5 minutes until kale wilts.
- Serve hot.

Nutrition per serving: 1 cup vegetables with 1 chicken thigh Calories – 374 | Fat – 19.3 g | Carbohydrate – 25.6 g | Fiber – 2.9 g | Protein – 24.7 g

58. Sticky Honey-Soy Chicken Wings

Total preparation time: 2 hr. 25 min | Yield: 6 to 8 servings
Ingredients

- Kosher salt and freshly ground black pepper
- 2 tbsps. extra-virgin olive oil
- 2 tbsps. butter
- ½ cup of honey
- Sesame seeds, for garnish
- 2 pounds chicken wings
- 1 cup of low sodium soy sauce,
- 1 tbsp. grated fresh ginger
- 2 tbsps. chopped fresh cilantro leaves
- 2 cloves garlic, minced ● ½ lemon, juiced

Directions

- Rinse chicken wings, dry pat. Remove tip and discard; split each wing in 2 parts. In a shallow bowl, put wings and pour over soy sauce, ginger, cilantro, garlic and lemon juice. Marinate well, refrigerated, for 2 hours.
- Marinade wings and pat dry; salt and pepper season. Melt butter in olive oil in a big, medium-high heat sauté pan. When the butter finishes foaming, add the honey and chicken wings and fry for about 5 mins. Continue cooking the wings, sometimes turning over to cover them as the glaze decreases. Cook until wings are sticky and baked. Garnish and serve sesame seeds.

59. One-Skillet Mediterranean Chicken Recipe with Tomatoes and Green Olives

Preparation Time: 10 mins | Cook Time: 15 mins | Total Time: 25 minutes
Ingredients:

- 4 boneless, skin chicken breasts of equal size
- 2 tbsps. minced garlic Salt and pepper
- 1 tbsp. dried oregano, divided
- Private Reserve extra virgin olive oil
- ½ cup of dry white wine
- 1 large lemon juice
- ½ cup of chicken broth
- 1 cup of finely chopped red onion
- 1 ½ cup of small-diced tomatoes
- ¼ cup of sliced green olives
- Handful of fresh parsley, stems removed, chopped Crumbled feta cheese, optional

Directions:

- Dry chicken breasts with a paper towel. Make three slits in the chicken breasts on each side.
- Garlic should be spread on both sides, and some garlic should be inserted into the incisions you formed. Season both sides of a chicken breasts with salt, pepper, and 12 tsp. dry oregano.
- 2 tbsp olive oil, heated over medium-high in a large cast iron skillet both sides of the chicken should be browned. Allow the white wine to reduce by 12 percent before adding the lemon juice and chicken broth. On top, sprinkling the remaining oregano. Turn the heat down to medium. Cover securely with foil or a lid. Cook for 10-15 minutes, flipping the chicken once (the internal temperature of the chicken should be around 165 degrees F.)
- Remove the lid and scatter the chopped onions, tomatoes, and olives on top. Cook for another 3 minutes, covered. Add the parsley and feta cheese last. Serve with light spaghetti, rice, or couscous as a dipping sauce. Take pleasure in it.

60. Skillet Chicken with Grapes and Caramelized Onions

Preparation Time: 15 mins | Cook Time: 50 mins | Yield: 4 servings

Ingredients:

For the caramelized onions

- 2 tbsps. butter
- 1 yellow onion, thinly sliced

For the chicken:

- ½ cup of flour
- ½ tsp salt
- ½ tsp chili powder
- ¼ tsp thyme
- ¼ tsp allspice
- 2 lbs. chicken thighs with skin (4-5)
- 2 tbsp. oil
- ¾ cup of dry red wine
- ½ cup of chicken broth
- 2 cups of red California grapes
- Parsley for topping

Directions:

- In a heavy pan, melt butter over medium-low heat to caramelize the onions. Cook onions for about 20 mins, stirring regularly. When the onions are a rich golden color, remove and put aside.
- Preheat oven to 400 degrees to make chicken. Combine rice, cinnamon, chili, thyme, allspice, and black pepper. Dredge each chicken in the flour mixture, shaking off the waste.
- Heat oil over medium heat in the same pan as onions. Add every piece of chicken skin-side down and fried until golden brown for a few mins, flip and cook for a few mins. Switch to a plate (if it's not completely baked, that's good – it'll finish in the oven – it's just getting browned on the outside).
- Turn the fire off and let oil cool off. Add the wine, it'll certainly bubble and sizzle! Attach broth and boil until

somewhat thickened. Add the onions and the chicken to the pan and bake 20 mins.

- Remove from the oven, add the strawberries, sauce and bake for another 5-10 mins. Serve with the green salad, bread, quinoa, rice, etc.

CHAPTER 4: PASTA

61. Shrimp Pasta Salad with Avocado

Preparation Time: 10 minutes | Cooking Time: 20 minutes | Servings: 4

Ingredients:

- 12 oz. fusilli pasta
- 1 lb. medium shrimp (peeled and deveined)
- 1 avocado (diced)
- 1-pint cherry tomatoes (halved)
- 1/2 red onion (thinly sliced)
- 1/4 cup chopped fresh parsley
- 1/4 cup chopped fresh basil
- 1/4 cup extra-virgin olive oil
- 2 tablespoonful red wine vinegar
- 1 tablespoonful Dijon mustard
- Salt and pepper, to taste

Directions:

- Cook the fusilli pasta according to package instructions until al dente. Drain and rinse under cold water to stop the cooking process. Set aside.
- In a large bowl, whisk together the olive oil, red wine vinegar, Dijon mustard, salt, and pepper to make the dressing.
- Add the cooked pasta, shrimp, avocado, cherry tomatoes, red onion, parsley, and basil to the bowl with the dressing. Toss gently until everything is coated in the dressing.
- Serve immediately or chill in the refrigerator until ready to serve.

Nutrition per serving: Calories: 485 | Total fat: 23g | Saturated fat: 3g | Cholesterol: 172mg | Sodium: 371mg | Total carbohydrate: 44g | Dietary fiber: 8g | Total sugars: 5g | Protein: 28g

62. Easy Mediterranean Pasta with Tuna and Tomatoes

Number of servings: 8

Ingredients:

- 16 ounces multigrain or whole-wheat fusilli spiral pasta
- 2 cans (14.5 ounces each) diced tomatoes with Italian seasonings, seasonings, with its liquid
- ½ cup brine-cured capers, drained
- 1 cup chopped fresh Italian flat leaf parsley
- 4 teaspoons finely grated lemon zest
- Salt to taste
- 2 tablespoons extra-virgin olive oil
- Pepper to taste
- ½ cup pitted, brine-cured black olives, quartered
- 2 cans (6 ounces each) water packed tuna, with its liquid its liquid
- 1 tablespoon minced fresh oregano
- 2 tablespoons fresh lemon juice

Directions:

- Cook the pasta. Retain about ½ cup of cooked pasta water and drain off the remaining water.
- Pour oil into a heavy skillet and heat over medium flame. When the oil is heated, add tomatoes, capers, olives, and retained pasta water and mix well.
- When the mixture begins to boil, add pasta and tuna and mix well.
- Lower the flame and cook for a couple of minutes. Break the tuna into bite-size chunks, as you stir.
- Add oregano, parsley, lemon juice, and lemon zest and stir. Add salt and pepper to taste. Serve hot.

Nutrition per serving: Calories – 274 | Fat – 6 g | Carbohydrate – 38.2 g | Fiber – 2.6 g | Protein – 17.7 g

63. Eyeball Pasta

Number of servings: 8
Ingredients:

- 4 slices soft, wholewheat bread, remove crusts (should weigh 2 ½ ounces after removing crusts), cubed
- 2 teaspoons olive oil
- 8 cloves garlic, finely chopped
- 12 ounces lean ground beef
- 12 ounces lean ground turkey
- 2 large eggs
- 6 tablespoons minced Italian flat leaf parsley, divided
- ½ teaspoon pepper
- 2 tablespoons low-sodium tomato paste
- 2 tablespoons raw honey
- 14 ounces whole wheat spaghetti
- 6 tablespoons 2% milk
- 2 white onions, finely chopped
- 6 tablespoons grated parmesan cheese
- 3 teaspoons Italian seasoning, divided
- 2 boxes (26 ounces each) unsalted chopped tomatoes
- 2 tablespoons balsamic vinegar
- ¼ cup chopped fresh basil
- ½ teaspoon red pepper flakes
- 14 ounces whole wheat spaghetti
- Salt to taste

Directions:

- Combine milk and bread in a bowl.
- Pour oil into a large skillet and heat over medium-high flame. Cook onions until light brown. Stir in garlic and sauté for 30 seconds. Turn off the heat.
- Transfer 1/3 of the onions into the bowl of bread. Also add in meat, salt, half of – parsley, pepper, and Italian seasoning. Mix until just incorporated. Make 1 inch balls of the mixture and place on a greased and foil-lined baking sheet.
- Set up the temperature of your oven to 425° F and preheat the oven. Bake the meatballs until they are not pink in the center.
- Cook pasta following the package directions.
- Combine the rest of the ingredients (except honey and basil) with the remaining onions in the skillet. Cook until thick.
- Add honey, basil, and meatballs and stir. Serve over pasta.

64. Whole Grain Pasta with Tomato Sauce, Grilled Vegetables, and Grated Parmesan Cheese

Preparation Time: 15 minutes | Cooking Time: 30 minutes | Servings: 4
Ingredients:

- 1 red bell pepper (seeded and sliced into strips)
- 1 small eggplant (sliced into rounds)
- 1 zucchini (sliced into rounds)
- 1/4 cup extra-virgin olive oil (divided)
- Salt and black pepper to taste
- 8 ounces whole grain pasta
- 2 cups tomato sauce
- 1/4 cup grated Parmesan cheese
- Fresh basil leaves for garnish

Directions:

- Preheat a grill or grill pan over medium-high heat. Toss the sliced red pepper, eggplant, and zucchini with 2 tablespoons of olive oil and season with salt and black pepper.
- Grill the vegetables for 5-7 minutes on each side, or until they are tender and slightly charred. Remove from heat and set aside.
- Cook the pasta according to package instructions until al dente. Drain and set aside.
- Heat the remaining 2 tablespoons of olive oil in a saucepan over medium heat. Add the tomato sauce and bring to a simmer.
- Add the grilled vegetables to the tomato sauce and stir to combine. Simmer for 5 minutes to allow the flavors to meld.
- Serve the pasta with the tomato and vegetable sauce, topped with grated Parmesan cheese and fresh basil leaves.

Nutrition per serving: Calories: 372 | Total Fat: 16.4g | Saturated Fat: 3.6g | Cholesterol: 7mg | Sodium: 617mg | Total Carbohydrates: 46.1g | Dietary; Fiber: 8.9g | Sugar: 11.3g | Protein: 13.7g

65. Spaghetti Nicoise

Preparation time: 30 mins – 1 hour | serves: 4-6
Ingredients:

- 350 g spaghetti
- 8 quail eggs
- 1 lemon
- 550 g tinned tuna in oil
- 60 g pitted and halved kalamata olives
- 100 g semi-dried tomatoes, halved lengthways
- 4 anchovy fillets, chopped into small pieces
- 3 tbsp baby capers, drained and rinsed
- 3 tbsp chopped flat-leaf (Italian) parsley

Direction:

- Cook the pasta in a quickly boiling salted water until al dente. Let it get hot, then drain and return. Meanwhile, lower the eggs into a cold water bath and cook for 4 mins (10 mins for hen eggs). Peel, rinse, cool, then rest. Cut eggs in two (or the hen eggs into quarters). Finely grind the lemon to give 1 tsp of grated zest. Then squeeze two tsp of lemon juice.
- Empty the tuna into a large bowl. Add olive oil, tomato quarters, anchovy fillets, lemon zest, capers, parsley and juice. Drop the spaghetti softly into the tuna. Garnish with the eggs and the parsley

66. Italian Mussels & Pasta

Number of servings: 8
Ingredients:

- 16 ounces whole-wheat linguine or spaghetti
- 4 large cloves garlic, chopped
- A large pinch of saffron, soaked in ¼ cup water
- 1 ½ cups dry white wine
- ½ teaspoon salt

- ½ cup chopped parsley
- ½ cup extra-virgin olive oil
- 2 cans (15 ounces each) crushed tomatoes with basil
- 4 pounds mussels, cleaned
- ½ teaspoon crushed red pepper
- Freshly ground pepper to taste
- 2 tablespoons finely grated lemon zest

Directions:
- Follow the directions on the package and cook the pasta. Drain and set aside in a large bowl. Cover the bowl.
- Pour oil into a large saucepan and heat over medium flame. When the oil is heated, add garlic and cook until light brown.
- Add tomatoes and the soaked saffron along with the water and stir. Cook until slightly thick, stirring often.
- Meanwhile, place mussels in a large pot. Pour wine into the pot. Place the pot over high flame. When the mixture begins to boil, lower the flame and cook covered, for about 5 – 6 minutes. If you find any unopened mussels, discard those.
- Place a fine wire mesh strainer over a bowl. Strain the mussel's mixture into the bowl. Pour the liquid into the simmering tomatoes. Add crushed red pepper, salt, and pepper and stir. Cook for a minute.
- Add half the sauce over pasta and toss well. Divide into 8 bowls. Divide mussels among the bowls. Pour remaining sauce over the mussels. Sprinkle parsley and lemon zest on top and serve

Nutrition per serving: Calories – 471 | Fat – 17 g | Carbohydrate – 55.6 g | Fiber – 9.2 g | Protein – 20.4 g

67. Spaghetti al Crudo

Preparation time: 15 minutes | serves: 4
Ingredients:
- 1 lb. Spaghetti
- 3 Tomato
- 4 fl. oz Olive oil
- 5 Anchovy fillets, pieces
- 4 tbsp Olive
- 2 oz. Basil
- 2 tbsp Capers
- 2 tbsp Tomato juice Pepper black ground, to taste

Directions:
- Put all the ingredients, except for spaghetti and basil, in a saucepan, cover with three spoons of olive oil - this is about 70 grams, mix, but do not heat. Try, salt and pepper.
- Bring the water to a boil in a large saucepan, add salt (a little less than usual, as anchovies will add an extra salty taste later) and put the pasta into it.
- Boil for about a minute less than what is indicated on the pack, to the state of al dente.
- While the pasta is boiling, place the stew-pan with the tomatoes and everything else on the saucepan with the pasta so that the steam heats them a bit and they are infused. When the paste is ready, drain the water, but do not completely pour it out.

- Mix the pasta with the ingredients of the sauce, adding a little water in which the pasta was boiled, if necessary so that the mixture does not turn out to be steep.
- Add the remaining olive oil and mix again. Add basil leaves in a saucepan and mix them with pasta. After that serve immediately.

Nutrition per serving: Calories: 115 Kcal | Fat: 7.7 g. | Protein: 6.2 g. | Carbs: 2 g

68. Simple Mediterranean Olive Oil Pasta

Preparation time: 10 mins Cook | Time: 9 mins | Total Time: 19 minutes
Ingredients:
- 1 lb. thin spaghetti
- ½ cup of Early Harvest Greek Extra Virgin Olive Oil (or Private Reserve Extra Virgin Olive Oil)
- 4 garlic cloves, crushed
- Salt 1 cup of chopped fresh parsley
- 12 oz. grape tomatoes, halved
- 3 scallions (green onions), top trimmed, both whites and greens chopped
- 1 tsp black pepper
- 6 oz. marinated artichoke hearts, drained
- ¼ cup of pitted olives, halved
- ¼ cups of crumbled feta cheese, more if you like
- 10-15 fresh basil leaves, torn Zest of
- 1 lemon Crushed red pepper flakes, optional

Direction:
- Cook thin spaghetti noodles according to package directions until al dente (mine took 6 minutes to cooks in plenty of boiling water with salt and olive oil).
- Heat the extra virgin olive oil in a big cast iron pan over medium heat when the pasta is almost done. Reduce a heat to low and season with a touch of salt and garlic. Cook for a total of 10 seconds, stirring often. Combine the parsley, tomatoes, and scallions in a mixing bowl. Cook for about 30 seconds over low heat, or until just warmed through.
- Remove the pasta from the heat, drain the cooking water, and return it to the saucepan. Toss in the hot olive oil sauce to cover well. Toss in the black pepper and toss one more to coat.
- Toss with the remaining ingredients one more time. Serve immediately in pasta bowls, topped with additional basil leaves and feta cheese if desired. Have fun!

69. Pesto Pasta with Chicken and Tomatoes

Preparation time: 15min | Cooking time: 15min | Servings: 6
Ingredients:
Pesto:
- 1 cup firmly packed fresh basil leaves
- 1/3 cup grated Parmesan cheese
- ¼ cup olive oil - 1 clove garlic
- 2 tablespoons sliced almonds, toasted

Pasta: -
- 12 oz. uncooked penne pasta (3 1/2 cups) (from 16-oz package)
- 3 cups Progresso™ chicken broth (from 32-oz carton)
- 2 cups shredded cooked chicken

- 2 cups halved cherry tomatoes
- ¼ cup julienned fresh basil leaves
- 3 tablespoons grated Parmesan cheese

Directions:
- In blender or food processor, place Pesto ingredients.
- Cover and process on medium speed about 3 minutes, stopping occasionally to scrape down sides with rubber spatula, until smooth. Set aside.
- In 4-quart saucepan, heat penne and broth just to boiling over high heat. Reduce heat to medium; cover and cook 8 to 10 minutes, stirring frequently, until al dente and liquid is almost absorbed. Remove from heat. Add pesto; stir in chicken and tomatoes; cook over medium 2 to 3 minutes or until thoroughly heated.
- Garnish with basil and 3 tablespoons Parmesan cheese.

Nutrition per serving: calories 480kcal | protein 27g | carbs 52g | fat 19g

70. Cheesy Spinach & Artichoke Stuffed Spaghetti Squash

Preparation time: 25min | Servings: 4

Ingredients:
- 1 (2 1/2 to 3 pound) spaghetti squash, cut in half lengthwise and seeds removed
- 3 tablespoons water, divided
- 1 (5 ounce) package baby spinach
- 1 (10 ounce) package frozen artichoke hearts, thawed and chopped
- 4 ounces reduced-fat cream cheese, cubed and softened
- ½ cup grated Parmesan cheese, divided
- ¼ teaspoon salt
- ¼ teaspoon ground pepper
- Crushed red pepper & chopped fresh basil for garnish

Directions:
- Place squash cut-side down in a microwave safe dish; add 2 tablespoons water. Microwave, uncovered, on High until tender, 10 to 15 minutes. (Alternatively, place squash halves cut-side down on a rimmed baking sheet. Bake at 400 degrees F until tender, 40 to 50 minutes.)
- Meanwhile, combine spinach and the remaining 1 tablespoon water in a large skillet over medium heat. Cook, stirring occasionally, until wilted, 3 to 5 minutes. Drain and transfer to a large bowl.
- Position rack in upper third of oven; preheat broiler.
- Use a fork to scrape the squash from the shells into the bowl. Place the shells on a baking sheet. Stir artichoke hearts, cream cheese, 1/4 cup Parmesan, salt and pepper into the squash mixture. Divide it between the squash shells and top with the remaining 1/4 cup Parmesan. Broil until the cheese is golden brown, about 3 minutes. Sprinkle with crushed red pepper and basil, if desired.

Nutrition per serving: calories 223kcal | protein 10g | carbs 23g | fat 10g | fiber 9g

71. Ravioli with Artichokes & Olives

Preparation time: 10min | Cooking time: 15min | Servings: 2

Ingredients:

- 2 (8 ounce) packages frozen or refrigerated spinach-and-ricotta ravioli
- ½ cup oil-packed sun-dried tomatoes, drained (2 tablespoons oil reserved)
- 1 (10 ounce) package frozen quartered artichoke hearts, thawed
- 1 (15 ounce) can no-salt-added cannellini beans, rinsed
- ¼ cup Kalamata olives, sliced
- 3 tablespoons toasted pine nuts
- ¼ cup chopped fresh basil

Directions:
- Bring a large pot of water to a boil. Cook ravioli according to package directions. Drain and toss with 1 tablespoon reserved oil; set aside.
- Heat the remaining 1 tablespoon oil in a large nonstick skillet over medium heat. Add artichokes and beans; sauté until heated through, 2 to 3 minutes.
- Fold in the cooked ravioli, sun-dried tomatoes, olives, pine nuts and basil.

Nutrition per serving: calories 454kcal | protein 15g | carbs 40g | fat 19g | fiber 13g

72. Mediterranean Pasta

Preparation time: 5 mins | Cook time: 15 mins | Total: 20 mins

Ingredients:
- 1 tbsp. kosher salt + 1 tsp, divided
- 6 ounce whole wheat angel hair pasta whole wheat spaghetti
- 4 cloves garlic
- 2 cups of grape tomatoes or cherry tomatoes
- 1 can quartered artichoke hearts
- 1 can whole pitted black olives
- 3 tbsps. good-quality olive oil
- 1/2 tsp ground black pepper
- -1/2 tsp crushed red peppers flakes
- 1/4 cup of freshly squeezed lemon juice about
- 1 lemon
- 1/4 cups of freshly grated Parmesan cheese
- 1/4 cup of fresh Italian parsley chopped

Directions:
- Bring the big saucepan of water to a boil with 1 tablespoon of salt in it. Cook a pasta until it is al dente (firm to the bite). Drain all except 12 cup of the pasta water.
- Prep your veggies and additional ingredients while the water boils and the pasta cooks: mince a garlic; halve the cherry tomatoes; drain and roughly cut the artichokes; drain and slice the olives in half. The dish moves rapidly as the veggies begin to cook, so be prepared.
- In the large pan, heat the olive oil over medium-high heat. Toss in the tomatoes, garlic, 1 teaspoon salt, pepper, and crushed red pepper flakes. Cooks, stirring frequently, for 1 to 2 minutes, or until the garlic is aromatic and the tomatoes have broken down and released some juices into the oil.
- Toss the spaghetti in the skillet to coat it. Combine the artichokes and olives in a bowl. Pour the lemon juice over

the spaghetti and toss to combine. Toss for another 1 to 2 minutes. If a pasta appears to be too dry, a dash of the leftover pasta water can be added to soften it up. Taste and season with salts and pepper to taste. Remove from a heat and top with Parmesan cheese and parsley. Toss once more, then eat.

73. Seafood Pasta

Preparation time: 25 minutes | serves: 4
Ingredients:

- 7 oz. Pasta
- 5 oz. Cream
- 4 oz. Shrimps
- 2 oz. Calamari
- 2 oz. Mussels
- 2 fl. oz. White dry wine
- 2 fl. oz. Tomato sauce
- 1 fl. oz. Olive oil
- 2 tsp Parmesan
- 1 tsp Green Basil
- 1 tsp Garlic

Directions:

- Fry seafood with garlic in olive oil.
- Add white wine, heavy cream, tomato sauce, salt, white ground pepper, and nutmeg.
- Mix with boiled pasta, add chopped basil. When serving, sprinkle with grated parmesan.

Nutrition per serving: Calories: 211 Kcal | Fat: 8.8 g. | Protein: 9.2 g. | Carbs: 22 g

74. Scoglio

Preparation time: 5 mins | Cook time: 47 mins | Total time: 52 mins | Yield: Makes 6 servings (1 serving: 2 cups)
Ingredients:

- 2 tbsps. olive oil
- 2 garlic cloves, crushed
- 1 (16-ounce) can whole Italian tomatoes
- Salt and freshly ground black pepper, as need
- 1 tsp Sicilian oregano (optional)
- 1 pound dry spaghetti
- 2 tbsps. + 2 tsp olive oil, divided
- 4-6 medium-size scallops
- ¼ tsp salt
- ¼ tsp pepper
- 8 medium-size peeled shrimp
- 1 spring fresh oregano
- 1 sprig fresh thyme
- 8 mussels
- 8 clams
- ½ cup of white wine

Directions:
MAKE SAUCE

- Heat oil in a saucepan. Cook a combination of garlic and oil, stirring. Put tomatoes into a bowl; split them up with clean hands. When garlic is browned, add tomatoes. Add salt and pepper.

- Simmer for 45 mins, adding water to prevent the sauce from thickening. The sauce should be dark red. If it turns brick red, it's too dense.

MAKE PASTA:

- Follow box instructions. Drain, reserving 1 cup of cooking water.
- Heat the 2 tsp oil in a skillet. Season scallops with salt and pepper, and fry until golden brown on either side. Remove and Separate.
- Cook shrimp before they are.
- Turn pink, for 1-2 mins then remove and reserve.
- Add reserved pasta water with oregano and thyme. Cook for 10 mins to make a soup, scraping the bottom of the pan to release the bits leftover from sautéing into the soup.
- When broth is ready, substitute mussels with 2 remaining tsp oil. Cook 2-3 mins, removing mussels until they open. Save. Repeat for clams, cooking 4 mins. Set back.
- Strain the broth and switch to the same bowl. Brown meat in oil over medium heat before alcohol burns off. Send scallops to the plate. Then add ½ cup of Pomodoro. Remove shrimp and a bit more sauce. Add spaghetti to the saucepan. Stir in sauce. Stir 2-3 mins and fold in clams and mussels. Serve instantly.

Nutrition per serving: 433 calories | fat 10.4g | saturated fat 1.6g |mono fat 6.1g | poly fat 1.6g | cholesterol 25mg | Protein 19g; carbohydrates 61g | sugars 2g | fiber 4g | Iron 4mg | sodium 491mg.

CHAPTER 5: FISH AND SEAFOOD

75. Skillet Salmon with Tomato Quinoa

Ingredients

- 2tsp canola oil
- 3cloves garlic, finely chopped
- 1 cup of cooked quinoa
- 3/4 cup of canned diced tomatoes
- 1/4tsp paprika Salt Pepper
- 1 cup of loosely packed baby spinach
- 2tbsp fresh basil, chopped
- 1salmon filet (3 ounces, skin removed)

Directions

- Preheat the oven to 425 degrees Fahrenheit.
- Heat oil in a shallow ovenproof skillet over medium heat. Cook, stirring constantly, for 1 minute, or until garlic is fragrant. Combine the quinoa, onions, and paprika in a mixing bowl. Salt and pepper to taste. Cook, stirring constantly, until thoroughly cooked. Stir in the spinach and basil to wilt them.
- Season the salmon with a generous amount of salt and pepper. On top of the quinoa mixture, position the salmon. Transfer to oven and roast for 8 to 12 minutes for medium rare, and 12 to 18 minutes for well cooked (the thicker your fillets, the longer it will take).
- Allow leftovers to cool fully before storing in the refrigerator in an airtight bag. NUTRITION PER SERVING 503 calories, 18 g fats (2 g saturated), 54 g carbs, 6 g sugar, 10 g fiber, 30 g protein.

76. Herby Fish with Wilted Greens & Mushrooms

Preparation time: 25min | Servings: 4

Ingredients:

- 3 tablespoons olive oil, divided
- ½ large sweet onion, sliced
- 3 cups sliced cremini mushrooms
- 2 cloves garlic, sliced
- 4 cups chopped kale
- 1 medium tomato, diced
- 2 teaspoons Mediterranean Herb Mix (see Associated Recipes), divided
- 1 tablespoon lemon juice
- ½ teaspoon salt, divided
- ½ teaspoon ground pepper, divided
- 4 (4 ounce) cod, sole, or tilapia fillets
- Chopped fresh parsley, for garnish

Directions:

- Heat 1 Tbsp. oil in a large saucepan over medium heat.
- Add onion; cook, stirring occasionally, until translucent, 3 to 4 minutes. Add mushrooms and garlic; cook, stirring occasionally, until the mushrooms release their liquid and begin to brown, 4 to 6 minutes.
- Add kale, tomato, and 1 tsp. herb mix. Cook, stirring occasionally, until the kale is wilted and the mushrooms are tender, 5 to 7 minutes. Stir in lemon juice and 1/4 tsp. each salt and pepper.

- Remove from heat, cover, and keep warm. -Sprinkle fish with the remaining 1 tsp. herb mix and 1/4 tsp. each salt and pepper. Heat the remaining 2 Tbsp. oil in a large nonstick skillet over medium-high heat.
- Add the fish and cook until the flesh is opaque, 2 to 4 minutes per side, depending on thickness. Transfer the fish to 4 plates or a serving platter. Top and surround the fish with the vegetables; sprinkle with parsley, if desired.

Nutrition per serving: calories 220kcal | protein 18g | carbs 11g | fat 11g | fiber 3g

77. Grilled Squid

Servings: 4
Ingredients:
For The Marinade

- 1 garlic clove, minced
- 3 tbsps. white or light miso paste
- 3 tbsps. sake
- 2 tsp mirin
- 1 tbsp. soy sauce
- 1 tbsp. oyster sauce
- 8 calamari, rinsed and dried

For The Slaw

- 2 tsp grated fresh ginger
- 1 ½ tsp cider vinegar
- Juice of 1 lime
- ½ tsp sugar
- Coarse salt, as need
- 3 tbsp. canola oil
- 5 celery stalks, halved and sliced into 2 ½-inch pieces
- 1 tart apple, such as Granny Smith, peeled and cut into matchsticks
- 2 scallions, halved and sliced into 2 ½-inch matchsticks
- ¾ cup of sunflower sprouts
- 1 serrano chile, halved, seeded, and thinly sliced crosswise
- 1 tsp black sesame seeds

Directions:

- In a medium-sized skillet, cook garlic, miso, sake, mirin, soy sauce, and oyster sauce for 3 mins, stirring periodically. Transfer to a bowl. Nice mildly.
- Tenderize the calamari by smashing it with a kitchen mallet. Cut the skin of the calamari, open it like a book. Lightly score at ¼ inch intervals. Add calamari to marinate for 20 mins.
- Mix ginger, vinegar, lime juice, cinnamon, and salt together. Add oil gently, whisking until emulsified.
- Preheat grill to medium-high. (When cooking on a barbecue, the coals are ready when the hand can be placed 5 inches above the grill for around 3 to 4 seconds.) Pour marinade off calamari and season sides with salt. Put calamari on grill and top with foil-lined weight. Cook the peppers until black. Split into ¾-inch-wide bits.
- Placed celery, apple, and scallions in a salad with the dressing (reserve remaining dressing for another use). Arrange on a platter. Cover with calamari, scatter with sesame seeds.

78. Curried Tilapia Brown Rice Bowl

Total Time: 10 mins | Yield: 1 serving
Ingredients:

- 1 tsp canola oil
- 1 carrot, diced
- 1 clove garlic, chopped
- ¼ cup of frozen peas
- 1 pounch of Chicken of the Tilapia Select Fillet in Yellow Curry Sauce.
- 1/8 tsp curry powder (optional)
- 1 cup of cooked hot brown rice
- Fresh mint (optional)
- 2 radishes, sliced (optional)

Direction:

- Heat oil medium-high in a 10-inch non-stick skillet. Add carrot and cook 3 mins.
- Add garlic and stir for 1 minute.
- Add peas, tilapia. Add 1/4 cup warm water to the Tilapia pouch and swish to get all the tasty sauce and pour into the oven. If needed, add curry powder. Cook until the peas are thawed, about 3 mins.
- Pour over rice and mint and radishes, if desired.

79. Salmon with Sorrel Sauce

Preparation time: 15 minutes | serves: 4
Ingredients:

- 1 lb. Salmon
- 10 oz Sorrel
- 5 fl. oz Sour cream
- 1 Onion 4 tbsp White dry wine
- 1.5 oz Butter Pepper black ground, to taste

Directions:

- Finely chop the onion and sorrel. Melted butter in a frying pan, add onion and fry until transparent. Then add sorrel and simmer for 4-5 minutes over medium heat under a closed lid. At this time, cut the fish into portions.
- We spread on a plate and tightly wrapped with cling film so that there is no escape to the air. Sent in a microwave at maximum power for 5 minutes.
- Add wine to the pan with sorrel and stew without a lid for 2-3 minutes, then add sour cream, salt, pepper and leave for another couple of minutes.
- Pour the prepared salmon into the sauce and serve it to the table!

Nutrition per serving: Calories: 114 | Kcal Fat: 9.7 g. | Protein: 1.6 g. | Carbs: 3.8 g

80. Mediterranean Fish Skillet

Ingredients:

- 1 large tomato, seeded and finely chopped
- 1 small green pepper, finely chopped
- 1 jalapeno pepper, seeded and minced
- 3 tbsps. minced fresh basil
- 3 tbsps. white wine or chicken broth
- 1 shallot, sliced
- 1 garlic clove, minced
- 1/2 tsp chili powder, divided
- 2 whitefish fillets (5 ounces every)
- 1 tbsp. olive oil

Directions:

- Set aside the tomato, peppers, basil, wine, shallot, garlic, and 1/4 teaspoon chili powder in a small bowl.
- The remaining chili powder should be sprinkled over the fillets. Cook fillets in oil for 4-5 minutes on each side or until fish flakes easily with a fork in a big pan over medium-high heat, adding tomato mixture during the final 3 minutes of frying.

81. Cabbage with Shrimps and Lemongrass

Preparation time: 25 minutes | serves: 4
Ingredients:

- 1 White cabbage
- 1 lb. Shrimps
- 4 fl. oz. Rice vinegar
- 1 Cilantro, bundle
- 1 White onion
- 2 oz. Ginger
- 4 fl. oz. Olive oil
- 2 tbsps. Soy sauce
- 4 Lemongrass
- 5 Garlic, cloves
- 2 Bay leaf

Directions:

- In a heated wok, fry the onion and ginger in olive oil.
- Add the chopped cabbage and simmer, stirring gently, until soft.
- Add soy sauce, finely chopped garlic, bay leaf, and sliced lemongrass.
- Simmer for 5-7 minutes, then add rice vinegar. Stir, stew for another couple of minutes, add shrimp and mix with cabbage.
- As soon as the shrimps are ready, sprinkle the contents of the wok with minced cilantro, stir and serve.

Nutrition per serving: Calories: 81 Kcal | Fat: 3.5 g. | Protein: 5 g. | Carbs: 8.8 g

82. Baked Clams Oreganata

Preparation time: 40 min | Yield: 1 dozen clams
Ingredients

- 1 dozen littleneck clams, scrubbed
- 1 cup of plain bread crumbs
- 2 cloves garlic, smashed and chopped
- 3 tbsps. finely chopped fresh oregano leaves
- 2 tbsps. finely chopped Italian parsley leaves
- Pinch crushed red pepper flakes
- Kosher salt
- 2 to 3 tbsps. extra-virgin olive oil
- ½ to ¾ cup of chicken stock

Directions:

- Heat the oven to 450 F.
- Place the clams in the oven at 200C for two to three mins or until the clams open. We want to transform the clams but not boil them.

- Using a butter knife carefully cut the clams, discarding the top shell. Take out the top half of the clam and put it back in the shell. That will make eating better.
- Preheat the oven, place the rack on the upper shelf.
- In a dish, combine the bread crumbs, garlic, parsley, and some cracked red pepper. Mix the olive oil with the onions. Attach chicken stock to make it wet. Taste the seasoning, add more salt if needed.
- Fill each clam with bread crumbs. Pack the bread crumbs down into the container. It will keep the clam moist.
- Spread clams on a sheet tray and apply about ½ cup of water. Moisture will help preserve the clams. Turn the oven on and place the bread crumbs under the broiler for 5-6 mins.

83. Gambas al Ajillo (Spanish Garlic Shrimp)

Number of servings: 12
Ingredients:
- 2 pounds large shrimp, peeled, peeled, deveined
- 1 cup extra virgin olive oil
- 2 teaspoons red pepper flakes
- 4 tablespoons dry sherry or dry white wine
- 1 cup chopped fresh parsley
- Kosher salt to taste
- 20 cloves garlic, peeled, chopped
- 2 teaspoons paprika
- Juice of a lemon
- Whole-wheat bread or crusty bread to serve

Directions:
- Dry the shrimp by patting with paper towels. Sprinkle salt over the shrimp.
- Pour oil into a large skillet and heat over medium flame. When the oil is hot but not smoking, add garlic and red pepper flakes and cook for a few seconds until the garlic is slightly brown in color.
- Stir in paprika and shrimp and cook for a few seconds until shrimp turns pink. This should happen in 3 – 4 minutes. Turn off the heat.
- Add sherry, parsley, and lemon juice and mix well. Divide into serving bowls and serve with bread.

Nutrition per serving: Without bread Calories – 249.5 | Fat – 19.2 g | Carbohydrate – 2.4 g | Fiber – 0.4 g | Protein – 16 g

84. Dilly Salmon

Preparation time: 10min | Grill time: 15min | Servings: 10
Ingredients:
- 1 cup Dijon mustard - 2/3 cup white wine or chicken broth
- 1/2 cup packed brown sugar
- 1/4 cup cider vinegar
- 3 tablespoons soy sauce
- 1 cup vegetable oil
- 1/2 cup minced fresh dill
- 1 teaspoon pepper
- 1 salmon fillet (1 inch thick and 3 pounds), cut in half widthwise

Directions:

- In a small bowl, whisk the mustard, wine, brown sugar, vinegar and soy sauce until well blended. Gradually whisk in oil. Stir in dill and pepper. Place salmon in a shallow glass dish. Pour 2 cups marinade over salmon.
- Cover and refrigerate for 1 hour. Cover and refrigerate remaining marinade for basting.
- Drain and discard marinade. Using long handled tongs, moisten a paper towel with cooking oil and lightly coat the grill rack. Place salmon skin side down on grill.
- Grill, covered, over medium-hot heat or broil 4 in. from the heat for 5 minutes. Baste with some of the reserved marinade. Grill or broil 7-9 minutes longer or until fish flakes easily with a fork, basting occasionally.

Nutrition per serving: calories 292kcal | protein 19g | carbs 7g | fat 3g

85. Seafood Gumbo

Preparation time: 20min | Cooking time: 30min | Servings: 24
Ingredients:
- 1 cup all-purpose flour
- 1 cup canola oil
- 4 cups chopped onion
- 2 cups chopped celery
- 2 cups chopped green pepper
- 1 cup sliced green onions
- 4 cups chicken broth
- 8 cups water
- 4 cups sliced okra
- 2 tablespoons paprika
- 1 tablespoon salt
- 2 teaspoons oregano
- 1 teaspoon ground black pepper
- 6 cups small shrimp, rinsed and drained, or seafood of your choice
- 1 cup minced fresh parsley
- 2 tablespoons Cajun seasoning

Directions:
- In a heavy Dutch oven, combine flour and oil until smooth. Cook over medium-high heat for 5 minutes, stirring constantly. Reduce heat to medium. Cook and stir about 10 minutes more or until mixture is reddish brown.
- Add the onion, celery, green pepper and green onions; cook and stir for 5 minutes. Add the chicken broth, water, okra, paprika, salt, oregano and pepper. Bring to boil; reduce heat and simmer, covered, for 10 minutes.
- Add shrimp and parsley. Simmer, uncovered, about 5 minutes more or until seafood is done.

Nutrition per serving: calories 166kcal | protein 10g | carbs 10g | fat 10g | fiber 2g

86. Charred Shrimp, Pesto & Quinoa Bowls

Preparation time: 25min | Cooking time: 0min | Servings: 4
Ingredients:
- ⅓ cup prepared pesto
- 2 tablespoons balsamic vinegar
- 1 tablespoon extra-virgin olive oi
- ½ teaspoon salt

- ¼ teaspoon ground pepper
- 1 pound peeled and deveined large shrimp (16-20 count), patted dry
- 4 cups arugula
- 2 cups cooked quinoa
- 1 cup halved cherry tomatoes
- 1 avocado, diced

Directions:
- Whisk pesto, vinegar, oil, salt and pepper in a large bowl. Remove 4 tablespoons of the mixture to a small bowl; set both bowls aside.
- Heat a large cast-iron skillet over medium high heat. Add shrimp and cook, stirring, until just cooked through with a slight char, 4 to 5 minutes. Remove to a plate.
- Add arugula and quinoa to the large bowl with the vinaigrette and toss to coat. Divide the arugula mixture between 4 bowls. Top with tomatoes, avocado and shrimp. Drizzle each bowl with 1 tablespoon of the reserved pesto mixture.

Nutrition per serving: calories 429kcal ;protein 30g ;carbs 29g ; fat 22g ; fiber 7g

87. Cherry Tomato Salad with Shrimps

Preparation time: 10 minutes | serves: 2
Ingredients:
- 11 oz. Cherry tomato
- 4 oz. Boiled shrimps, peeled
- 1oz Green basil
- 1 fl. oz. Olive oil lb. Mussels
- 1 glass White dry wine
- 8 oz. Cheese
- 8 oz. Cream
- 1/2 Onions head
- 2 tbsps. Olive oil
- 1 tbsp. Parsley, chopped
- 2 Garlic, cloves Pepper black ground, to taste

Directions:
- Cherry tomatoes cut in half and add peeled shrimp. Add the chopped basil leaves.
- Add olive oil, add salt and pepper.

Nutrition per serving: Calories: 66 Kcal | Fat: 4.9 g. | Protein: 3.8 g. | Carbs: 2.1 g

88. Oven-Poached Lemon Butter Cod

Preparation time: 10min | Cooking time: 20min | Servings: 6
Ingredients:
- 6 5-ounce pieces of cod, about 2 lbs.
- 1/4 pound butter
- 1 small or ½ large lemon
- 1/2 cup dry vermouth
- 1 clove garlic, minced
- 1 tablespoon minced parsley
- ½ teaspoon salt
- ¼ teaspoon pepper
- Optional: extra lemon slices for garnish

Directions:
- Preheat the oven to 400 degrees. Spray a 9 x 9 pan with nonstick spray then arrange cod pieces inside of it.

- Melt butter in a small saucepan (or microwave in a bowl) then squeeze in the lemon juice. Add the vermouth, chopped parsley, garlic, salt, and pepper to the butter mixture and mix until combined.
- Pour the butter mixture over the cod fillets -Bake until the cod is opaque and flakes easily with a fork, approximately 15-20 minutes. Drizzle with butter to serve, and top with a lemon wedge if desired.

Nutrition per serving: calories 328kcal | protein 35g | carbs 3g | fat 5g

89. Fish Stew with Potatoes and Tomatoes
Servings: 4

Preparation time: 15 minutes | cooking time: 30 minutes
Ingredients:
- 1 lb. firm white fish (such as cod or halibut), cut into chunks
- 4 medium-sized potatoes, peeled and cut into small cubes
- 1 onion (chopped)
- 3 garlic cloves (minced)
- 1 red bell pepper (chopped)
- 1 can (14 oz.) diced tomatoes
- 1 cup vegetable or chicken broth
- 1 tablespoonful olive oil
- 1 teaspoonful smoked paprika
- 1 teaspoonful dried thyme
- Salt and pepper, to taste
- Chopped fresh parsley, for garnish

Directions:
- Heat the olive oil in a large pot over medium heat. Add the onions and garlic and cook until the onions are translucent, about 3-4 minutes.
- Add the potatoes and red bell pepper to the pot and cook for another 3-4 minutes.
- Add the diced tomatoes, broth, smoked paprika, thyme, salt, and pepper. Stir to combine.
- Bring the mixture to a boil, then reduce the heat to low and let it simmer for 10 minutes, or until the potatoes are tender.
- Add the fish chunks to the pot and let it cook for another 5-7 minutes, or until the fish is cooked through.
- Garnish with chopped fresh parsley and serve hot.

Nutrition per serving: Calories: 298kcal| Fat: 6g | Saturated Fat: 1g | Cholesterol: 69mg | Sodium: 468mg | Carbohydrates: 28g | Fiber: 5g | Sugar: 7g | Protein: 33g

90. Seafood Couscous Paella

Number of servings: 4
Ingredients:
- 4 teaspoons extra virgin olive oil
- 2 cloves garlic, minced
- 1 teaspoon fennel seeds
- ½ teaspoon freshly ground pepper
- 2 cups unsalted, canned diced tomatoes with their juice
- 8 ounces small shrimp, peeled, deveined
- 8 ounces bay scallops, discard tough muscles
- 1 cup whole-wheat couscous
- 2 medium onions, chopped

- 1 teaspoon dried thyme
- ½ teaspoon salt
- A large pinch of saffron threads, threads, crumbled
- ½ cup vegetable broth

Directions:
- Place a large saucepan over medium flame. Add oil and let it heat. Once the oil is hot, add onion and sauté until translucent.
- Stir in thyme, garlic, fennel seeds, saffron, pepper, and salt and stir for a few seconds until you get a nice aroma.
- Add tomatoes and broth and stir. When the mixture begins to boil, lower the flame and cook covered for a couple of minutes.
- Raise the heat to medium flame. Add scallops and cook for a couple of minutes.
- Stir in the shrimp. Once shrimp is cooked for 2 minutes, add couscous and stir. Turn off the heat. Let it sit covered for 5 minutes. Uncover and fluff the mixture with a fork

Nutrition per serving: 1 ½ cups Calories – 403 | Fat – 6.8 g | Carbohydrate – 60.3 g | Fiber – 9.6 g | Protein – 26.6 g

91. Roasted Fish with Vegetables

Preparation time: 35min | Cooking time: 20min | Servings: 4
Ingredients:
- 1 pound fingerling potatoes, halved lengthwise
- 2 tablespoons olive oil
- 5 garlic cloves, coarsely chopped
- ½ teaspoon sea salt
- ½ teaspoon freshly ground black pepper
- 4 5 to 6-ounce fresh or frozen skinless salmon fillets
- 2 medium red, yellow and/or orange sweet peppers, cut into rings
- 2 cups cherry tomatoes
- 1 ½ cups chopped fresh parsley (1 bunch)
- ¼ cup pitted kalamata olives, halved
- ¼ cup finely snipped fresh oregano or 1 Tbsp. dried oregano, crushed
- 1 lemon

Directions:
- Preheat oven to 425 degrees F. Place potatoes in a large bowl. Drizzle with 1 Tbsp. of the oil and sprinkle with garlic and 1/8 tsp. of the salt and black pepper; toss to coat. Transfer to a 15x10-inch baking pan; cover with foil. Roast 30 minutes.
- Meanwhile, thaw salmon, if frozen. Combine, in the same bowl, sweet peppers, tomatoes, parsley, olives, oregano and 1/8 tsp. of the salt and black pepper. Drizzle with remaining 1 Tbsp. oil; toss to coat.
- Rinse salmon; pat dry. Sprinkle with remaining 1/4 tsp. salt and black pepper. Spoon sweet pepper mixture over potatoes and top with salmon. Roast, uncovered, 10 minutes more or just until salmon flakes. Remove zest from lemon. Squeeze juice from lemon over salmon and vegetables. Sprinkle with zest.

Nutrition per serving: calories 422kcal | protein 32g | carbs 31g | fat 18g | fiber 5g

92. Lemon Salmon with Garlic and Thyme

Number of servings: 8
Ingredients:
- 8 salmon fillets (5 – 6 ounces each)
- Kosher salt to taste
- 1 teaspoon dried thyme
- Extra virgin olive oil, as required
- 2 whole lemons, grate the rind, cut the lemon into thin round slices
- 10 cloves garlic, peeled, crushed
- Freshly ground pepper to taste

Directions:
- Set up the temperature of your oven to 400° F and preheat the oven. Keep the salmon in a baking dish. Pour oil over the fillets. Sprinkle salt, pepper, lemon zest, and thyme over the fillets.
- Place lemon slices and garlic over the salmon. Place the baking dish in the oven and bake for about 20 minutes or until it flakes easily when pierced with a fork.

Nutrition per serving: Calories – 356 | Fat – 23 g | Carbohydrate – 0 g | Fiber – 0 g | Protein – 32 g

93. Creamy Salmon Soup

Preparation time: 30 minutes | serves: 6
Ingredients:
- 1 lb. Cream of 10%
- 1 lb. Potato
- 11 oz. Salmon
- 10 oz. Tomato
- 7 oz. Leek
- 5 oz. Carrot
- 1 Greens, bunch
- 2 tbsps. Olive Oil Pepper black ground, to taste

Directions:
- Cut leek rings, rub carrots with a grater. Peeled potatoes cut into small cubes or cubes.
- Cut the salmon into cubes. Peel the tomatoes and cut into cubes. If the skin is badly removed, dip the tomatoes for a few seconds in boiling water.
- In a saucepan fry onions and carrots in olive oil. Add tomatoes and fry slightly.
- Pour 1 liter of water, bring to a boil. When the water boils, add potatoes, salt to taste, cook for 5-7 minutes. Then add the salmon and pour in the cream.
- Boil until potatoes are ready (3-5 minutes).

Nutrition per serving: Calories: 115 Kcal | Fat: 7.7 g. | Protein: 6.2 g. | Carbs: 2 g.

94. Cabbage with Shrimps and Lemongrass

Preparation time: 25 minutes | serves: 4
Ingredients:
- 1 White cabbage
- 1 lb. Shrimps
- 4 fl. oz. Rice vinegar
- 1 Cilantro, bundle
- 1 White onion
- 2 oz. Ginger
- 4 fl. oz. Olive oil

- 2 tbsps. Soy sauce
- 4 Lemongrass
- 5 Garlic, cloves
- 2 Bay leaf

Directions:

- In a heated wok, fry the onion and ginger in olive oil. Add the chopped cabbage and simmer, stirring gently, until soft.
- Add soy sauce, finely chopped garlic, bay leaf, and sliced lemongrass. Simmer for 5-7 minutes, then add rice vinegar.
- Stir, stew for another couple of minutes, add shrimp and mix with cabbage. As soon as the shrimps are ready, sprinkle the contents of the wok with minced cilantro, stir and serve.

Nutrition per serving: Calories: 81 Kcal Fat: 3.5 g. | Protein: 5 g. | Carbs: 8.8 g

CHAPTER 6: VEGETARIAN MAINS
95. Vegetable Soup

Preparation time: 10 minutes | Cooking time: 30 minutes | Servings: 4

Ingredients:

- 2 tablespoons olive oil
- 1 onion (chopped)
- 3 garlic cloves (minced)
- 2 medium carrots (chopped)
- 2 celery stalks (chopped)
- 1 small zucchini (chopped)
- 1 small yellow squash (chopped)
- 4 cups vegetable broth
- 1 can (14 oz) diced tomatoes
- 1 teaspoonful dried oregano
- 1 teaspoonful dried basil
- Salt and black pepper to taste
- Fresh parsley (chopped, for serving)

Directions:

- Heat the olive oil in a large pot over medium heat. Add the onion and cook until softened, about 5 minutes.
- Add the garlic, carrots, celery, zucchini, and yellow squash. Cook for another 5-7 minutes, stirring occasionally, until the vegetables start to soften.
- Pour in the vegetable broth and diced tomatoes, and bring the mixture to a boil.
- Reduce the heat to low and simmer the soup for 20-25 minutes, or until the vegetables are tender.
- Add the dried oregano and basil, and season the soup with salt and black pepper to taste.
- Serve hot, garnished with fresh parsley.

96. Vegan Mediterranean Wraps

Preparation time: 30 minutes | Total Time: 30 minutes

Ingredients:

- 1 medium cucumber
- ½ tsp (+ a couple pinches) of salt divided
- 1 medium tomato diced
- ¼ red onion diced
- ¼ green pepper diced
- 4 tbsps. chopped kalamata olives
- 1 jar (540 grams / 19 oz.) chickpeas
- 200 grams (7 oz.) vegan yogurt (I used soy)
- 2 tbsps. chopped fresh dill
- 1 clove of garlic minced
- 1 tbsp. lemon juice
- Pepper as needed
- 2 cups of (112 grams) chopped lettuce
- 4 large tortillas

Direction:

- Half the cucumber should be grated and seasoned with a bit of salt. Place it in the colander over a bowl to drain while you chop the rest of your vegetables. Half of the cucumber should also be diced. Cucumber, tomato, red onion, green pepper, and black olives are chopped and mixed together.

- Place the chickpeas in a bowl after draining and rinsing them. Use your hands or a fork to smash them.
- Squeeze as much water as you cans out of the shredded cucumber. Toss the grated cucumber with the vegan yogurt, dill, garlic, lemon juice, and a pinch of salt & pepper in a mixing bowl.
- Toss the crushed chickpeas with 3 tbsps. tzatziki and 12 tsp salt and pepper. Mix thoroughly.
- A handful of lettuce, smashed chickpeas, chopped mixed veggies, and a couple dollops of tzatziki go inside the wraps. You may toast the final wraps in a dry pan over medium-high heat if you want to.

97. Quinoa Vegetable Soup

Preparation Time: 15 mins | Cook Time: 45 mins | Total Time: 1 hour

Ingredients:

- 3 tbsps. extra virgin olive oil
- 1 medium yellow or white onion, chopped
- 3 carrots, peeled and chopped
- 2 celery stalks, chopped
- 1 to 2 cups of chopped seasonal vegetables, like zucchini, yellow squash, bell pepper, sweet potatoes or butternut squash
- 6 garlic cloves, pressed or minced
- ½ tsp dried thyme
- 1 large can (28 ounces) diced tomatoes
- Scant 1 cup of quinoa, rinsed well in a fine mesh colander (use less for a lighter, more broth-y soup)
- 4 cups of (32 ounces) vegetable broth
- 2 cups of water 1 tsp salt, more as need
- 2 bay leaves Pinch red pepper flakes
- Freshly ground black pepper
- 1 can great northern beans or chickpeas, rinsed and drained
- 1 cup of or more chopped fresh kale or collard greens, tough ribs removed
- 1 to 2 tablespoon of lemon juice, as need
- Optional garnish: freshly grated Parmesan cheese

Direction:

- In the big Dutch oven or soup pot, heat the olive oil over medium heat. Add the chopped onion, cabbage, celery, seasonal vegetables, and a touch of salt until the oil is shimmering. Cooks, stirring often, for 6 to 8 minutes.
- Garlic and thyme can be included now. Cook for 1 minute, stirring constantly. Cooks for a few more minutes, stirring often, after adding the diced tomatoes with their juices.
- Mix the quinoa, broth, and water in a mixing bowl. 1 tsp salt, 2 bay leaves, and a pinch of red pepper flakes are added to the pot. Season with freshly ground black pepper as need. Raise the heat to high and bring the mixture to a boil, then reduce heat to low and sustain a gentle simmer.
- Drop the cap after 25 minutes and stir in the beans and chopped greens. Continue to cook, stirring occasionally, for another 5 minutes or until the greens have softened to your taste.

- Remove the bay leaves after removing the pot from the sun. 1 tsp lemon juice 1 tsp lemon juice 1 tsp lemon juice 1 tsp lemon juice 1 tsp lemon juice 1 Season with more salt, pepper, and/or lemon juice if required until the flavors are vibrant. (Depending on your vegetable broth and personal tastes, you can need up to 12 tsp more salt.) If desired, divide into bowls and finish with grated Parmesan cheese.

98. Ultimate Gazpacho

Preparation Time: 25 minutes | Cook Time: 0 minutes | Total Time: 25 minutes

Ingredients:

- 2 ½ pounds ripe red tomatoes
- 1 small Vidalia or sweet yellow onion, peeled and cut into rough 1" chunks
- 1 small cucumber, peeled and seeded
- 1 medium red bell pepper, cored and seed
- ¼ cups of fresh basil leaves, + extra for garnish
- 1 large garlic clove, peeled
- ¼ cup of extra-virgin olive oil
- 2 tbsps. sherry vinegar
- ¾ tsp fine sea salt
- Freshly ground black pepper

Directions:

- Place your mixer tray, a medium serving bowl, and a small bowl on the counter to cook your vegetables. Break the tomatoes into rough 1'' bits after removing the cores. Place around a quarter cup of the juicy tomato seeds in a little bowl (we'll use them as a garnish later). Half of the tomato chunks should go into the mixer, and the other half should go into the serving bowl. In a mixer, mix all of the onion chunks.
- Remove only a quarter of the cucumber. Place the piece in the small bowl after finely chopping it. The remaining cucumber can be sliced into rough 1" chunks and divided between the blender and the serving bowl. Remove about a quarter of the bell pepper, finely chop it, and place it in the small bowl. The remaining bell pepper can be sliced into rough 1" chunks and divided between the blender and the serving bowl.
- Connect the basil, ginger, olive oil, vinegar, cinnamon, and about 10 twists of black pepper to the blender. Secure a lid and blend, starting on low and gradually rising to high rpm, for around 2 minutes, or until the mixture is fully smooth.
- Fill the blender halfway with the contents of the serving bowl (the leftover cabbage, cucumber, and bell pepper chunks). Place a cap on the blender and blend for 10 to 20 seconds, or until the ingredients are broken up into tiny fragments. Stop here if you choose smaller pieces, or mix a bit longer if you choose larger ones.
- Toss the garnishes in a small bowl with a pinch of salt, stir, and store in the fridge. Allow at least 2 hour, and up to 24 hours, for the soup to chill. Taste before serving and season with more salt (I often add another 14 tsp) and/or black pepper if needed. To eat, split the soup into small bowls or cups of and top with the cucumber and bell pepper that have been set aside. Serve with a light sprinkle of pepper and a few tiny or broken basil leaves on top. Protected and refrigerated leftover servings hold well for 3 to 4 days.

99. White Bean Soup with Orange Slices and Olive Oil

Preparation time: 15min | Cooking time: 30min | Servings: 8

Ingredients:

- 4 large carrots, sliced thin
- 5 celery sticks, sliced thin
- 1 large onion, sliced thin
- 1 cup extra virgin olive oil
- 1/2 tsp dried oregano
- 1 bay leaf - 3 slices orange (skin and flesh)
- 2 tbsp. tomato paste
- 15 ounces cannellini (white) beans 4 cans
- 2 cups water

Directions:

- Sauté carrots, celery, and onion in olive oil on medium heat until soft.
- Add oregano and bay leaf.
- Add orange slices and tomato paste. Sauté for 2 minute.
- Add Cannellini beans, 2 cans with liquid, 2 cans drained. Add 2 cups water.
- Simmer for 30-40 minutes until soup thickens, stirring occasionally.

Nutrition per serving: calories 324kcal | protein 5g | carbs 17g | fat 27g | fiber 4g

100. Cilantro-Lime Cauliflower Rice

Prep Time: 5 mins | Cooking Time: 1 min | Number of Servings: 5

Ingredients:

- 1 medium to large head cauliflower, broken into florets
- 2 tablespoons olive oil
- ¼ teaspoon kosher salt
- 1 cup chopped fresh cilantro
- Juice of 1 lime

Directions:

- Place a steamer basket in the cooker pot and add 1 cup of water. Put the cauliflower florets into the steamer basket.
- Secure the lid and cook on high pressure for 1 minute, using a quick release at the end of the cooking time. Select cancel and open the lid carefully.
- Transfer the cauliflower to a plate. Carefully drain the water from the pot, wipe the pot dry, and put it back in the cooker.
- Select sauté and adjust to low. Heat the olive oil in the pot until the display reads hot. Add the cooked cauliflower and break it up with a potato masher.
- Season with the salt, add the cilantro and stir gently while the cauliflower rice heats.

Nutrition per Serving:

Calories: 202 | Total fat: 14g | Saturated fat: 2g | Cholesterol: 0mg | Carbohydrates: 19g | Fiber: 8g | Protein: 6g

101. Bacon Honey Sprouts

Prep Time: 5 mins| Cooking Time: 8-10 mins| Number of Servings: 2-3

Ingredients:

- 1 tablespoon honey
- 4 slices of bacon, chopped
- ½ cup of water
- Sea salt as needed
- 4 cup Brussels sprouts, chopped

Directions:

- Add the bacon in the pot; cook for 4-5 minutes to crisp it.
- Add the sprouts and cook for 4-5 more minutes. Pour the water.
- Close the pot and cook for 2 minutes.
- Open the pot and serve the prepared dish warm! Add some salt if needed.

Nutrition per Serving:
Calories – 57Fat – 8.5g|Carbohydrates – 6g|Fiber – 1g|Protein – 4g

102. Mediterranean Vegan Cabbage Soup

Preparation Time: 15 mins | Cook Time: 35 minutes | Total Time: 50 minutes

Ingredients:

- Extra virgin olive oil
- 2 medium-sized onions, sliced into half-moons
- 2 garlic cloves, minced
- 2 large carrot, peeled and sliced into rounds
- 2 russet potatoes, scrubbed clean and sliced into ¼ inch-thick rounds
- 1 ½ lb. green cabbage (about ½ head of cabbage), cored and chopped
- Kosher salt and pepper
- 1 tbsp. organic ground cumin
- 1 tsp sweet Spanish paprika
- ½ tsp ground coriander
- ¼ tsp ground turmeric Bay leaf
- 1 cup of tomato sauce
- 6 to 7 cup of low-sodium vegetable broth Zest + juice of 1 lemon
- ½ cup of fresh dill Pinch crushed red pepper (optional)

Direction: Stove-Top Cabbage Soup

- 2 tbsps. extra virgin olive oil, heated in a large Dutch oven or heavy saucepan until shimmering but not smoking, combine the onions, garlic, carrots, potatoes, and chopped cabbage in a large mixing bowl.
- Sauté the veggies for a few minutes, or until they're almost soft. Add the remainder of the spices and bay leaf after seasoning with salt and pepper.
- Cook for a few minutes more, tossing often. Combine the tomato sauce and broth in a mixing bowl. Raise a heat to high and bring the soup to a boil for 5 minutes, then reduce to low and partially cover the pot.
- Cook, stirring occasionally, for 30 to 40 minutes, or until veggies are soft.
- Finally, add the fresh dill, lemon zest, and lemon juice (or your choice of fresh herb.) Place in serving dishes.

Crock Pot Cabbage Soup

- In a bottom of a 6-quart crock pot like this one, layer carrots, potatoes, cabbage, onions, and garlic.
- Season with kosher salts and freshly ground black pepper. Combine the spices, bay leaf, tomato sauce, and broth in a large mixing bowl. To combine, stir everything together.
- Cooks on LOW for 7 to 8 hours or HIGH for 4 hours in a covered crock pot (or slow cooker). Mixing should be done on a regular basis.
- Unplug the crock pot when the soup is done. Combine the lemon zest, lemon juice, and fresh dill in a mixing bowl.
- Place the soup in serving bowls.

Instant Pot Cabbage Soup

- In an instant pot, combine all of the ingredients except the lemon juice, lemon zest, and fresh dill.
- Lock the lid, lock the lid, and set the timer for 15 minutes on high, then allow the pot cool naturally (another 15-20 minutes.) Remove the cover and mix in the lemon zest, lemon juice, and fresh dill when it's done. Serve immediately in serving bowls.
- If desired, sauté the veggies first in the instant pot with little extra virgin olive oil before cooking.
- Drizzle a drizzle of Early Harvest extra virgin olive oil over the cabbage soup once it's been transferred to serving bowls.
- Add the sprinkle of red pepper flakes if you want it spicy. Serve with warm pita bread or a crusty whole wheat bread of your choice. Have fun!

103. Chinese cabbage with Mint and Green Peas

Preparation time: 5 minutes | serves: 4

Ingredients:

- 1/2 Chinese cabbage
- 4 oz. Green pea
- 1 Chili pepper
- 1 Fresh mint, bundle
- 2 tbsps. Sesame oil
- 1 tbsp. Rice vinegar
- 1 tbsp. Soy sauce

Directions:

- Heat the wok and pour in the sesame oil, and then the soy sauce with vinegar.
- Add chopped green peas, fry for 30 seconds, then add noodles of chopped cabbage and fry for one more minute. Add the mint, chopped chili peppers and mix.
- Turn off the heat and cover with a lid. Let it brew for a couple of minutes and serve.

Nutrition per serving: Calories: 77 Kcal Fat: 5.7 g. | Protein: 2 g. | Carbs: 5.9 g

104. Asparagus Lemon Flank

Prep Time: 5 mins| Cooking Time: 2 mins| Number of Servings: 2

Ingredients:

- 2 tablespoons lemon juice
- ¼ pound Asparagus
- 1 cup of water
- 1 teaspoon olive oil

Directions:

- Trim the asparagus and remove the woody parts.

- Add some lemon juice and olive oil over the asparagus then toss to combine.
- Switch on the pot after placing it on a clean and dry platform.
- Pour the water into the pot. Arrange the trivet inside it; arrange the asparagus over the trivet.
- It will take 8-10 minutes for natural pressure release.
- Open the pot and serve warm. Enjoy it with your loved one!

Nutrition per serving: Calories – 38| Fat – 2.5g| Carbohydrates – 2.8g| Fiber – 1g| Protein – 2g

105.   Vegetable Couscous

Yield: 4
Ingredients:
- ¼ cup of cooking oil
- 1 large onion, cut into thin slices
- 4 carrots, cut into thin slices
- 1 fennel bulb, cored and cut into 1-inch pieces
- 1 eggplant (¾ pound), cut into ½-inch pieces
- 4 minced cloves garlic
- 1 jalapeño pepper, includes seeds and ribs, cut into thin slices
- ¼ cup of tomato paste
- 2 tsp ground coriander
- 1 ½ tsp caraway seeds
- 2 ¼ tsp salt
- ¼ tsp fresh-ground black pepper
- 5 ½ cups of water
- 15-ounce drained and rinsed chickpeas
- 1 1/3 cups of couscous

Directions:
- Heat oil with low heat in a large saucepan. Add cabbage, carrots, fennel, garlic, and jalapeño. Cook, wrapped, about 10 mins to soften the vegetables. Tomato paste, coriander, caraway seeds, 2 salt tbsps., and black pepper. Cook 1 minute, stirring.
- Add 3 1⁄2 cups of sugar, then simmer. Reduce heat and cook about 15 mins, uncovered, until vegetables are tender. Add chickpeas and cook 2 mins longer.
- Meanwhile, in a medium saucepan, boil the remaining 2 cups of water. Add 1⁄4 tsp of salt and couscous. Cover. Cover. Remove the pot and let the couscous stand for 5 mins. Fluffing with a fork. Serve the broth over the couscous.

106.   Ratatouille

Prep Time: 25 mins| Cooking Time: 6 mins| Number of Servings: 2
Ingredients:
- 1 small eggplant, chopped
- Kosher salt
- 2 tablespoons oil, divided
- 1 small onion, chopped
- 1 garlic clove, minced
- 1 tablespoon mashed roasted garlic
- 1 zucchini, chopped
- 1 yellow summer squash, chopped

- 1 green bell pepper, seeded and chopped
- ¼ cup dry white wine
- ½ cup Vegetable Stock or water
- 2 basil leaves
- ½ teaspoon herbes de Provence
- Freshly ground black pepper
- 1 (14-ounce) can crushed tomatoes with their juices

Directions:
- In a colander set over a medium bowl, sprinkle salt on the eggplant, toss to coat, and let drain.
- Preheat pot till hot, add 1 tablespoon of oil to the pot. Add the onion and sauté until softened, 4 to 5 minutes. Add the minced garlic and roasted garlic and cook until fragrant, 1 minute.
- Add the zucchini, squash, and bell pepper and cook until softened, 4 to 5 minutes. Add the wine and deglaze the pot, scraping up any browned bits from the bottom and allowing the mixture to reduce by half, about 2 minutes. Carefully transfer the mixture to a large bowl and set aside.
- Heat the remaining 1 tablespoon of oil in the pot. Add the eggplant and brown, stirring frequently, 2 to 3 minutes. Press cancel.
- Return the vegetables to the pot, stir in the stock, basil, and herbes de Provence, and season with salt and pepper. Stir well, and then add the tomatoes and their juices.
- Secure the lid and cook on high pressure for 6 minutes, then allow the pressure to naturally release for 5 minutes.
- Stir the contents of the pot and let simmer until thickened, about 5 minutes.
- Serve sprinkled with chopped basil and grated Parmesan or vegan cheese.

Nutrition per Serving: Calories: 360| Total fat: 15g| Saturated fat: 2g| Cholesterol: 0mg| Carbohydrates: 46g| Fiber: 18g| Protein: 12g

107.   Mediterranean Cabbage Soup

Number of servings: 3
Ingredients:
- 1 tablespoon extra-virgin olive oil
- ½ cup sliced fennel, retain the fronds to garnish
- 1 teaspoon minced garlic
- ¼ teaspoon salt or to taste
- ½ can (from a 15 ounces can) unsalted diced tomatoes with garlic, oregano, and basil
- ½ can (from a 15 ounces can) cannellini beans, rinsed
- ½ teaspoon chopped fresh oregano
- ½ cup chopped carrots
- ¼ cup chopped onions
- ¼ teaspoon ground coriander
- 3 cups low sodium vegetable broth
- ¾ pound cabbage, chopped
- 1 teaspoon sugar
- Grated lemon zest, to garnish
- Pepper to taste

Directions:

- Pour oil into a soup pot and place the pot over medium-high flame. When the oil is heated, add fennel, carrots, and onion and sauté until the onion turns pink.
- Stir in garlic, salt, and coriander and cook for a few seconds until you get a nice aroma in the air.
- Stir in tomatoes and broth. When the mixture begins to boil, lower the flame and add in the cabbage.
- Let it simmer until the cabbage is soft. Add sugar, beans, and oregano and cook for another 5 minutes.
- Ladle into soup bowls. Garnish with lemon zest and fennel fronds and serve.

Nutrition per serving: Calories – 205 | Fat – 5.5 g | Carbohydrate – 31 g | Fiber – 9.6 g | Protein – 6.2 g

108. Zucchini Soup

Preparation time: 15min | Cooking time: 30min | Servings: 4 Ingredients:

- 2 tablespoon olive oil
- 1 small onion, finely chopped
- 2 garlic cloves, minced
- 4 medium zucchini (1 ½ to 2 pounds), skin on, ends trimmed, halved lengthwise, and sliced
- 3 cups vegetable or chicken broth, or more as desired for a thinner texture
- ¼ cup raw cashews
- 1 teaspoon kosher salt
- ¼ teaspoon ground black pepper
- 2 tablespoons fresh lemon juice
- 2 tablespoons chopped fresh herbs (dill, basil, or parsley work great), plus more for garnish

Directions:

- Heat the oil in a large pot over medium-high heat. Add the onion and saute for 4-5 minutes, until softened. Add the garlic, and stir for another minute.
- Add the zucchini, broth, cashews, salt, and pepper, and bring to a boil. Turn the heat down to low, cover, and simmer for about 15 to 20 minutes, or until the zucchini is tender.
- Add the chopped herbs and lemon juice to the soup. Then use an immersion blender (stick blender) to blend the soup until smooth, or transfer the soup in batches to a high-powered blender, and blend for just 15-30 seconds, until smooth.
- Ladle portions of the zucchini soup into bowls and garnish with a drizzle of olive oil and fresh herbs.

Nutrition per serving: calories 167kcal | protein 5g | carbs 13g |; fat g | fiber g

109. Vegan Lentil Soup

Preparation time: 20min | Cooking time: 40min | Servings: 6
Ingredients:

- 2 tablespoons extra-virgin olive oil
- 1 ½ cups chopped yellow onions
- 1 cup chopped carrots
- 3 cloves garlic, minced
- 2 tablespoons no-salt-added tomato paste
- 4 cups reduced-sodium vegetable broth

- 1 cup water
- 1 (15 ounce) can no-salt-added cannellini beans, rinsed
- 1 cup mixed dry lentils (brown, green and black)
- ½ cup chopped sun-dried tomatoes in oil, drained
- ¾ teaspoon salt
- ½ teaspoon ground pepper
- 1 tablespoon chopped fresh dill, plus more for garnish
- 1 ½ teaspoons red-wine vinegar

Directions:

- Heat oil in a large heavy pot over medium heat. Add onions and carrots; cook, stirring occasionally, until softened, 3 to 4 minutes. Add garlic and cook, stirring constantly, until fragrant, about 1 minute. Add tomato paste and cook, stirring constantly, until the mixture is evenly coated, about 1 minute.
- Stir in broth, water, cannellini beans, lentils, sun-dried tomatoes, salt and pepper. Bring to a boil over medium-high heat; reduce heat to medium-low to maintain a simmer. Cover and simmer until the lentils are tender, 30 to 40 minutes.
- Remove from heat and stir in dill and vinegar. Garnish with additional dill, if desired and serve.

Nutrition per serving: calories 272 kcal | protein 13g | carbs 72g | fat 7g | fiber 9g

110. Brown Rice with Chinese Vegetable Stir-Fry

Prep Time: 10 mins | Cooking Time: 15 mins | Number of Servings: 2
Ingredients:

- 3 tablespoons sesame oil, divided, plus more for greasing
- ¾ cup long-grain brown rice
- ¾ cup water, plus 3 tablespoons Kosher salt
- 1 tablespoon cornstarch
- 2 garlic cloves, crushed
- 1½ teaspoons peeled minced fresh ginger, divided
- 1 cup broccoli florets
- ½ cup julienned carrots
- ¾ cup snow peas, trimmed
- 3 fresh shiitake mushrooms, sliced
- ¼ cup drained sliced water chestnuts
- 2 to 3 tablespoons low-sodium soy sauce
- ¼ cup chopped onion

Directions:

- Coat the inside of the pressure cooker pot with sesame oil. Put the pot in the cooker.
- Add the rice and ¾ cup of water and season with salt. Secure the lid and cook on high pressure for 15 minutes, then allow the pressure to naturally release for 5 minutes. Open the vent at the top and remove the lid.
- While the rice is cooking, prepare the vegetables. In a large bowl, stir together the cornstarch, garlic, ½ teaspoon of ginger, and 2 tablespoons of sesame oil until combined and the cornstarch is dissolved. Add the broccoli, carrots, snow peas, mushrooms, and water chestnuts and toss to lightly coat.

- Heat the remaining 1 tablespoon of sesame oil in a wok over medium heat. Increase the heat to medium-high and add the vegetables. Cook for 2minutes, tossing constantly to prevent burning.
- Stir in the soy sauce and remaining 3 tablespoons of water. Add the onion and remaining 1 teaspoon of ginger and season with salt. Cook, stirring constantly, until the vegetables are tender but still crisp, 1 to 2 minutes.
- Divide the brown rice between two plates and top with the stir-fried vegetables.

Nutrition per serving: Calories: 618| Total fat: 23g| Saturated fat: 3g| Cholesterol: 0mg| Carbohydrates: 94g| Fiber: 9g| Protein: 10g

111. Tomato and White Bean Soup

Preparation time: 10 minutes | cooking time: 30 minutes | Servings: 6

Ingredients:
- 2 tablespoonful olive oil
- 1 onion (chopped)
- 3 garlic cloves (minced)
- 2 carrots (peeled and chopped)
- 2 celery stalks (chopped)
- 1 can (14 oz) diced tomatoes
- 4 cups vegetable broth
- 1 can (14 oz) white beans (rinsed and drained)
- 1 teaspoonful dried rosemary
- Salt and black pepper to taste
- Fresh basil (chopped, for serving)

Directions:
- Heat the olive oil in a large pot over medium heat. Add the onion and cook until softened, about 5 minutes.
- Add the garlic, carrots, and celery. Cook for another 5-7 minutes, or until the vegetables start to soften.
- Pour in the diced tomatoes and vegetable broth. Bring the mixture to a boil.
- Stir in the white beans, dried rosemary, and season with salt and black pepper to taste.
- Reduce the heat and simmer for 15-20 minutes, or until the vegetables are tender.
- Serve hot, garnished with fresh basil.

Nutrition per serving: Calories: 148 | Total Fat: 4.6g | Saturated Fat: 0.6g | Sodium: 610mg | Total Carbohydrates: 22g | Dietary Fiber: 6g | Sugar: 6g; Protein: 7g

112. Bell Pepper Vegetarian Omelet

Preparation time: 5 mins | Cook time: 10 mins Total time: 15 mins

Ingredients:
- 4 large eggs
- 1 tbsp. olive oil
- 1/2 medium onion, diced, optional
- 1 red bell pepper, thinly chopped
- 1 green bell pepper, thinly chopped
- 1 tbsp. unsalted butter (or margarine)
- Kosher salt, as need Freshly
- ground black pepper, as need
- 1/2 tsp garlic powder, optional

Directions:
- Collect the required ingredients.
- Crack eggs into a shallow mixing bowl and whisk them together vigorously with a fork to incorporate as much air as possible. Make a reservation.
- Heat olive oil in a nonstick skillet or omelet pan over medium heat. If using, add the diced onion and cook for 3 to 5 minutes.
- Cook, stirring sometimes, for 1 to 2 minutes, or until the bell peppers are slightly tender. Switch the heat off.
- Take onions and peppers out of the pan with a slotted spoon, leaving the oil behind. Mix the vegetables with the pounded eggs that have been set aside.
- Wipe the skillet clean with multiple paper towels before replacing it over medium-low heat.
- Add a butter and swirl it around in the pan to make sure it covers the entire rim.
- Pour in the egg mixture and season as need with salt and pepper, as well as the garlic powder, if using.
- Tilt the pan when lifting the omelet's sides to allow the uncooked center to flow out to the edges. This allows the eggs to cook more quickly and uniformly.
- Cook your vegetable omelet until the bottoms of the eggs are firm but not orange.
- Flip it over with a rubber spatula and cook for another 1 to 2 minutes before switching to a pan. Alternatively, fold the omelet in half and slide it onto a plate from the tray. The inside of the container should be moist but not fresh.
- Take pleasure in it.

CHAPTER 7: BEANS AND GRAINS

113. Southern Beans and Greens

Prep Time: 10 mins | Cooking Time: 10 mins | Number of Servings: 2

Ingredients:

- 1 tablespoon oil
- ½ yellow onion, diced
- 2 garlic cloves, minced
- 1 cup Chicken Stock
- ½ pound dried black-eyed peas
- 2 cups chopped Swiss chard or kale
- 1½ teaspoons red pepper flakes
- 2 fresh thyme sprigs or ½ teaspoon dried thyme
- ½ tablespoon kosher salt
- ¼ teaspoon freshly ground black pepper
- 1 tablespoon apple cider vinegar
- 1 to 2 teaspoons hot sauce (optional)

Directions:

- Add the oil to the pot, heat until hot, and add the onion. Cook, stirring often, for 2 minutes, or until softened. Add the garlic and cook, stirring, until fragrant, about 1 minute.
- Add the stock, peas, Swiss chard, red pepper flakes, thyme, salt, and pepper. Deglaze the pot by scraping all the flavorful brown bits up off the bottom of the pot with a wooden spoon, and then mix well.
- Cover the pot and cook on high heat for 10 minutes
- Pour in the vinegar and hot sauce (if using). Adjust seasoning if desired. Serve.

Nutrition per serving: Calories: 385 | Total fat: 8g | Saturated fat: 1g | Cholesterol: 0mg | Carbohydrates: 77g | Fiber: 32g | Protein: 31g

114. Grilled Chicken Caesar Salad with Whole Grain Croutons

Preparation Time: 15 minutes | Cooking Time: 15 minutes | Servings: 4

Ingredients:

- 2 boneless, skinless chicken breasts
- 2 tablespoonful of olive oil
- 1/2 teaspoonful garlic powder
- Salt and pepper, to taste
- 1 head of romaine lettuce (washed and chopped)
- 1/2 cup whole grain croutons
- 1/4 cup grated Parmesan cheese
- 1/4 cup Caesar dressing
- 1 lemon (sliced)

Directions:

- Preheat a grill or grill pan to medium-high heat.
- Season the chicken breasts with olive oil, garlic powder, salt, and pepper.
- Grill the chicken for 6-7 minutes on each side, or until fully cooked through. Let it rest for 5 minutes before slicing into strips.
- While the chicken is cooking, prepare the salad. In a large bowl, combine the chopped romaine lettuce, whole grain croutons, grated Parmesan cheese, and Caesar dressing. Toss to combine.

- Divide the salad into 4 bowls and top each with the sliced grilled chicken.
- Squeeze lemon juice over the salad and serve immediately.

Nutrition per serving: Calories: 330 | Protein: 27g | Fat: 20g | Carbohydrates: 10g | Fiber: 3g | Sugar: 2g

115. Fava Beans with Jasmine Rice Recipe

Preparation Time: 10 mins| Cook Time: 30 mins| Total Time: 40 mins| Servings: 4 servings

Ingredients

- 1 medium onion, chopped
- 4 garlic cloves, chopped
- 1 tbsp. (or more) olive oil
- 3 sprigs thyme leaves, fresh
- ½ cups of Fava beans, shelled
- 1 cup of Jasmine rice
- ½ tsp salt
- 2 cups of (add more) chicken stock (homemade or a good-quality store-bought)

Directions:

- Saute the onion and garlic in a big, medium-heat frying pan until the onions tend to soften and the mixture is fragrant.
- Reduce heat to low and add Fava beans, rice jasmine, salt, and chicken stock. Cook, lid askew, until rice is soft. Keep adding chicken stock if needed.
- When the rice is soft, reduce heat a little and cook until a golden crust appears on the rice rim. Control closely and don't burn rice. Add small quantities of chicken stock as needed. Using a spatula to search the rice rim. When golden, it raises effortlessly and stays together.
- Makes four servings.

116. White Bean Soup

Preparation time: 10min | Cooking time: 25min | Servings: 6

Ingredients:

- 1 tablespoon olive oil
- 1 large onion chopped
- 2 garlic cloves minced
- 2-3 large carrots chopped
- 2-3 celery rib chopped
- 6 cups vegetable broth
- 1 teaspoon dried thyme
- ½ teaspoon oregano
- 1 teaspoon salt
- ½ teaspoon black pepper
- 3 15-ounces canned white beans drained and rinsed
- 2 cups baby spinach
- Fresh parsley finely chopped, for serving
- Grated parmesan cheese for serving

Directions:

- In a large pot or saucepan, heat olive over medium high heat. Add onions and cook until onions are translucent, about 3-5 minutes. Add the garlic, carrots, celery, thyme, oregano, salt and pepper, and cook for an additional 2-3 minutes.
- -Add vegetable broth and beans, bring to a boil, reduce heat and simmer for 15 minutes to combine all of the flavors together. -Stir in the spinach and continue to simmer until the spinach wilts, about 2 minutes
- -Remove from heat, sprinkle fresh parsley and grated parmesan cheese, if desired, and serve immediately.

Nutrition per serving: calories 295kcal | protein 17g | carbs 52g | fat 3g

117. Slow-Cooker Quinoa with Arugula

Preparation time: 15min | Cooking time: 3h | Servings: 6

Ingredients:

- 2 ¼ cups unsalted vegetable stock
- 1 ½ cups uncooked quinoa, rinsed
- 1 cup sliced red onions (from 1 onion)
- 2 garlic cloves, minced (about 2 teaspoons)
- 1 (15.5 ounce) can no-salt-added chickpeas (garbanzo beans), drained and rinsed
- 2 ½ tablespoons olive oil
- ¾ teaspoon kosher salt
- 2 teaspoons fresh lemon juice (from one lemon)
- ½ cup drained, chopped roasted red bell peppers (from jar)
- 4 cups baby arugula (about 4 ounces)
- 2 ounces feta cheese, crumbled (about 1/2 cup)
- 12 pitted kalamata olives, halved lengthwise
- 2 tablespoons coarsely chopped fresh oregano

Directions:

- Stir together the stock, quinoa, onions, garlic, chickpeas, 1 1/2 teaspoons of the olive oil, and 1/2 teaspoon of the salt in a 5- to 6- quart slow cooker.
- Cover and cook on LOW until the quinoa is tender and the stock is absorbed, 3 to 4 hours.
- Turn off the slow cooker. Fluff the quinoa mixture with a fork. Whisk together the lemon juice and remaining 2 tablespoons olive oil and 1/4 teaspoon salt.
- Add the olive oil mixture and red bell peppers to the slow cooker; toss gently to combine. Gently fold in the arugula.
- Cover and let stand until the arugula is slightly wilted, about 10 minutes. Sprinkle each serving evenly with the feta cheese, olives, and oregano.

Nutrition per serving: calories 352kcal | protein 12g | carbs 46g | fat 7g | fiber 13g

118. Kidney Bean Curry

Preparation time: 5 mins | Cook time: 30 mins

Ingredients:

- 1 tbsp. vegetable oil
- 1 onion, finely chopped
- 2 garlic cloves, finely chopped
- thumb-sized piece of ginger, peeled and finely chop
- 1 small pack coriander, stalks finely chopped, leaves roughly
- shredded
- 1 tsp ground cumin
- 1 tsp ground paprika
- 2 tsp garam masala
- 400g can chopped tomatoes
- 400g can kidney beans, in water
- cooked basmati rice, to serve

Directions:

- In the big frying pan, heat the oil over low-medium heat. Cook, stirring occasionally, until the onion has softened and begun to color. Cook for another 2 minutes, and coriander stalks are fragrant.

- Add the spices to the pan and simmer for another minute, or before it smells fragrant. Put the chopped tomatoes and kidney beans, along with their water, to a boil.
- Reduce the heat to low and cook for 15 minutes, Or until the curry has thickened. Season with Salts and pepper as need, then serve with basmati Rice and coriander leaves.

119.   Italian Artichoke and Green Bean Casserole

Number of servings: 5
Ingredients:
- ¾ pound cut fresh green beans
- ½ medium onion, chopped
- 1 ½ cans (14 ounces each) water packed artichoke hearts, drained, chopped
- Cayenne
- Cayenne pepper to taste
- ½ cup seasoned whole-wheat breadcrumbs
- 3 tablespoons olive oil
- 1 clove garlic, minced
- ¼ cup minced fresh parsley
- Pepper to taste
- ½ cup grated parmesan cheese, divided
- Salt to taste

Directions:
- Set up the temperature of your oven to 350° F and preheat the oven.
- Place a pot, half-filled with water over high flame. When water begins to boil, add green beans and cook for about 2 – 3 minutes, until the beans are crisp as well as tender.
- Drain the beans in a colander.
- Place a pot over medium flame. Add oil and let it heat. Once the oil is heated, stir in the onion and cook until the onion turns pink.
- Stir in garlic and cook for 50 – 60 seconds. Now add the beans into the pot. Also add breadcrumbs, 6 tablespoons cheese, artichoke hearts, cayenne pepper, parsley, salt, and pepper. Mix well and turn off the heat.
- Add all the contents of the pot into a baking dish. Top with remaining cheese.
- Place the baking dish in the oven and bake until the cheese is light brown

Nutrition per serving: ¾ cup Calories – 207 | Fat – 10 g | Carbohydrate – 22 g | Fiber – 3 g | Protein – 8 g

120.   Mediterranean Plant Protein Power Bowl

Preparation Time: 10 minutes | Cook Time 15 minutes | Total Time 25 minutes
Ingredients:
- 1 cup of quinoa uncooked
- 2 cups of vegetable broth
- 2 cups of spinach
- 1/2 cup of cherry tomatoes
- 1/4 cup of kalamata olives sliced
- 1/4 cup of hummus

- 1/2 cucumber sliced
- 1/4 red onion thinly sliced
- 1/2 avocado diced
- 2 tbsps. olive oil
- 1/2 lemon juiced
- 1 tsp red wine vinegar dill optional

Direction:
- In the large saucepan on the stove, combine the quinoa and vegetable broth. Bring to a boil, then turn down to a low heat. Cooks for another 10 minute on low heat, covered (until majority of cooking liquid has been absorbed by quinoa). Turn off the heat.
- In the large mixing bowl, combine spinach leaves, cherry tomatoes, olives, hummus, cucumber, red onion, avocado, and quinoa.
- Drizzle olive oil, lemon juice, and red wine vinegar over the top.
- Add fresh chopped dill and season with salt and pepper (to taste) (if desired)

121.   Spinach & Bean Burrito Wrap

Preparation Time: 20 minutes | Total Time: 20 minutes
Ingredients
- 6 cups of baby spinach loosely packed
- 15 ounces black beans can and rinsed and drained
- 1 1/2 cups brown rice cooked
- 1/2 cup of romaine lettuce hearts chopped
- 1/2 cup of cheddar cheese grated, reduced-fat
- 1/2 cup of salsa (recipe), optional Pico de Gallo
- 6 tbsp Greek yogurt fat-free kosher or sea salt as need
- 6 whole grain wrap or tortillas, 8 inch

Directions:
- Preheat the oven to 300 degrees to warm the tortillas. When cooking the ingredients, stack tortillas, seal in foil, and put on a baking sheet to warm for 15 minutes.
- Put the spinach in a foods processor and rotate until it's finely diced, or dice the leaves with a knife. Heat a big skillet over medium-high heat, then add the black beans and spinach. Heat for 3 minutes, or until spinach is wilted.
- Distribute the spinach and bean mixture equally in the center of the wraps (leaving about 2" on one end for folding), 1/4 cup rice to each cover, lettuce, cheese, salsa, and Greek yogurt evenly across wraps. On the sides, fold the wraps over and under.

Nutrition per serving: 1wrap | Calories: 282kcal | Carbohydrates: 50g | Proteins: 13g | Fat: 5g | Cholesterol: 3mg | Sodium: 560mg | Fiber: 5g | Sugar: 3g

122.   Mediterranean Chicken Quinoa Bowl

Number of servings: 2
Ingredients:
- ½ pound boneless, skinless chicken breasts, trimmed
- 1/8 teaspoon pepper
- 1/8 cup
- 1/8 cup slivered almonds
- 2 small cloves garlic, crushed
- 1/8 cup pitted, chopped kalamata olives
- ½ cup diced cucumber

- 1 tablespoon finely chopped parsley
- 1/8 teaspoon salt
- ½ jar (from a 7 ounces jar) roasted red peppers, rinsed
- 2 tablespoons extra-virgin olive oil, divided
- ½ teaspoon paprika
- 1/8 teaspoon crushed red pepper
- ¼ teaspoon ground cumin
- 1 cup cooked quinoa
- 1/8 cup finely chopped red onion
- 1/8 teaspoon crumbled feta cheese

Directions:

- Place the rack in the upper third position in the oven. Set up your oven to broil mode and preheat it to high heat.
- Place a sheet of aluminum foil on a baking sheet. Season the chicken with salt and pepper and place it on the baking sheet.
- Place the baking sheet in the oven and let the chicken broil for about 7 – 8 minutes. Turn the chicken over and broil for another 7 – 10 minutes or until the internal temperature of the chicken in the meatiest part shows 165° F on a meat thermometer.
- Take out the chicken from the oven and place it on your cutting board. Let it cool for a few minutes. Cut into slices.
- Mix together quinoa, red onion, and olives in a bowl and divide it into 4 serving bowls.
- Blend together peppers, 1 tablespoon oil, garlic, and spices in a blender until smooth.
- Divide the chicken, cucumber, feta, and parsley among the bowls. Drizzle red pepper sauce on top and serve.

Nutrition per serving: 3 ounces chicken with ½ cup quinoa and ¼ cup sauce.
Calories – 519 | Fat – 26.9 g | Carbohydrate – 34.1 g | Fiber – 4.2 g | Protein – 34.1 g

123. Black Bean-Quinoa Buddha Bowl

Number of servings: 2
Ingredients:

- 1 ½ cups cooked or canned black beans, rinsed, drained
- ½ cup hummus
- ½ medium avocado, peeled, pitted, diced
- ¼ cup chopped fresh cilantro
- 1 1/3 cups cooked quinoa
- 2 tablespoons lime juice
- 6 tablespoons pico de gallo

Directions:

- Follow the instructions on the package of quinoa and cook quinoa. Measure out 1 1/3 cups of quinoa and add into a bowl. Add black beans and stir. Divide the mixture into two serving bowls.
- To make dressing: Whisk together hummus and lime juice in a bowl. Add a little water if you want a thinner dressing.
- Divide and drizzle the dressing over the bean mixture.
- Place avocado and pico de gallo on top. Garnish with cilantro and serve.

Nutrition per serving: Calories: 500 | Fat: 16 g | Carbohydrates: 74 g | Fiber: 20 g | Protein: 20 g

124. Lentil Soup

Preparation time: 10min | Cooking time: 1h | Servings: 6
Ingredients:

- 1 onion, chopped
- ¼ cup olive oil
- 2 carrots, diced
- 2 stalks celery, chopped
- 2 cloves garlic, minced
- 1 teaspoon dried oregano
- 1 bay leaf
- 1 teaspoon dried basil
- 1 (14.5 ounce) can crushed tomatoes
- 2 cups dry lentils
- 8 cups water
- ½ cup spinach, rinsed and thinly sliced
- 2 tablespoons vinegar
- salt to taste - ground black pepper to taste

Directions:

- In a large soup pot, heat oil over medium heat. Add onions, carrots, and celery; cook and stir until onion is tender. Stir in garlic, bay leaf, oregano, and basil; cook for 2 minutes.
- Stir in lentils, and add water and tomatoes. Bring to a boil. Reduce heat, and simmer for at least 1 hour. When ready to serve stir in spinach, and cook until it wilts. Stir in vinegar, and season to taste with salt and pepper.

Nutrition per serving: calories 349kcal | protein 18g | carbs 48g | fat 10g

CHAPTER 8: LAMB, PORK, AND BEEF

125. Herb-Roasted Boneless Leg of Lamb

Preparation time: 20 mins | Total: 3 hrs. | Yield: Makes 4 to 6 servings
Ingredients:

- 1 (5-lb.) boneless leg of lamb, rolled and tied
- 3 ½ tsp kosher salt, divided
- 2 tsp freshly ground black pepper, divided
- ¼ cup of loosely packed fresh rosemary leaves
- ⅔ cup of loosely packed fresh flat-leaf parsley leaves
- ¼ cup of loosely packed fresh thyme leaves
- 2 shallots, coarsely chopped
- 6 garlic cloves
- 1 tbsp. fresh lemon juice
- 10 tbsps. olive oil, divided
- 2 pounds small new potatoes

Directions:

- Rub salt into lamb. Salt and 1 tsp. pepper; let stand 1 hour.
- Pulse food processor 4 to 5 times or until finely chopped. Add the parsley and next four ingredients and pulse to finely cut. Add 6 Tbsp. Drizzle olive oil and pulse until smooth, scraping down sides as needed. Rub mixture over lamb; put in a large roasting pan. Let stand 30 mins.
- Bake at 450°. Put in potatoes and remaining tsp. salt, 1 tsp. pepper, and 4 Tbsp. oil, put potatoes around lamb in skillet.

- Bake for an hour or until a meat thermometer inserted into the thickest section reads 125° (rare). Let lamb rest, cover with foil, and let stand 15 mins before slicing.
- Dice half of the lamb and put it in a 2 (2-cup of) section in your storage tub. Serve lamb and potatoes with juices.
- Peel the middle of the potatoes for a pretty show.

126. Oven Roasted Pork Tenderloin

Prep Time: 10 mins | Cook Time: 30 mins | Total Time: 40 mins | Servings: 4
Ingredients:
- 1.4 lb. pork tenderloin
- Salt and Pepper
- 1 tbsp. Dijon mustard
- Herb Mixture
- 1.5 tbsp. olive oil
- 3 large cloves garlic chopped
- 1 tbsp. Italian seasoning
- ½ tsp coarse sea salt

Directions:
- Heat the oven to 350 F.
- Dijon Mustard: Put the tenderloin in the oven-safe bowl. Season the pork tenderloin with salt and pepper. Rub the Dijon mustard on the tenderloin.
- Herb mixture: In a small bowl, blend olive oil, chopped garlic, Italian seasoning and salt.
- Cover the tenderloin with the herb mixture on top on both sides, except the bottom.
- Roast at 350F for 30 mins. Then the internal temperature can exceed at least 145 F or 160 F (for white looking tenderloin). Leave in the oven for 5 mins. Cut and serve.

Nutrition per serving: Calories 246| Fat 11g| Cholesterol 103mg| Sodium 416mg|; Potassium 648mg; Protein 33g; Calcium 34mg; Iron 2.1mg

127. Spiced Beef Pilaf

Total time: 35 mins | Serves: 2 people
Ingredients:
- 250g beef mince
- 1 onion
- 1 garlic clove
- 1 tsp ground cumin
- 1 cinnamon stick
- 1 tsp ground turmeric
- 1 tsp coriander seeds
- 2 tomatoes
- 50g dried apricots
- 150g bulgar wheat
- 1 chicken stock cube
- 50g peppery salad leaves
- 1 tbsp. olive oil
- Sea salt
- Freshly ground pepper
- 500ml boiling water

Directions:
- Have a big pan on the stovetop. Chop up the beef and throw in the olive oil, salt and pepper. Get in there with the wooden spoon. Fry for 3-4 mins before browned.

- Finely chop the onion and garlic clove. Add 1 tsp per cumin, turmeric and coriander seeds and the cinnamon stick. Keep cooking, stirring regularly.
- When the stew simmers, loosely chop the tomatoes and apricots. Line them up.
- Add one stock cube to 500ml boiling water. Stir well until dissolved.
- Pour the bulgur wheat into the pan and add stock. Stir all ingredients together. Then reduce heat to a gentle simmer. Cook until wheat is soft and fluffy, about 15 mins.
- Take out the pan from the heat and allow to steam for five mins, with the lid on. Taste and add seasoning if needed.

128. Slow Cooker Beef Bourguignon

Preparation Time: 20 Mins | Cook Time: 9 Hours | Total Time: 9 Hours 20 Mins | Servings: 6 People
Ingredients:
- 5 slices finely chopped bacon
- 3 pounds boneless beef chuck cut in to 1 inch cubes
- 1 cup of red cooking wine
- 2 cups of chicken broth
- ½ cup of tomato sauce
- ¼ cup of soy sauce
- ¼ cup of flour
- 3 garlic cloves finely chopped
- Tbsp. thyme finely chopped
- 5 medium carrots sliced
- 1 pound baby potatoes
- 8 ounces fresh mushrooms sliced
- Fresh chopped parsley for garnish

Direction:
- Cook bacon until crispy in a skillet. Placed bacon in slow cooker. Season beef with the salt, pepper and sear on either side for 2-3 mins. Move beef to the slow cooker.
- Connect the red wine to the skillet. Slowly reduce and boil and add chicken broth, tomato sauce, and soy sauce. Slowly add the flour. Add the sauce to the slow cooker
- Add onions, garlic, and carrots to the slow cooker. Be sure to stir regularly and cook at low until the beef is tender for 8-10 hours or high for 6-8 hours.

Nutrition per serving: 6 Calories 181kcal| Carbohydrates22g |Protein7g| Fat8g | Saturated Fat3g | Cholesterol12mg | Sodium1062mg| Potassium646mg |Fiber3g |Sugar2g |Vitamin A199IU |Vitamin C27mg |Calcium31mg |Iron2mg

129. Vegetable Beef Soup

Preparation time: 20 minutes | Cook time: 1 hour 10 minutes | Total time: 1 hour 30 minutes
Ingredients:
- 1 1/2 lbs. beef stew meat
- 2 1/2 Tbsp. olive oil, divided Salt and freshly ground black pepper
- 1 3/4 cups of chopped yellow onion (1 large)
- 1 1/4 cups of peeled and chopped carrots (3 medium)
- 1 cup of chopped celery
- 1 1/2 tbsp. minced garlic
- 8 cups of low-sodium beef broth or chicken broth

- 2 cans diced tomatoes
- 1 1/2 tsp dried basil
- 1 tsp dried oregano
- 1/2 tsp dried thyme
- 1 lb. red , chopped into 3/4-inch cubes
- 1 1/2 cups of (5 oz.) chopped green beans (trim ends first)
- 1 1/2 cups of frozen corn
- 1 cup of frozen peas 1/3 cup of chopped fresh parsley

Directions:
- In the big pot, heat 1 tbsp. olive oil over medium-high heat.
- Dry the beef with paper towels, season with salt and pepper, and then brown half of it in the pot for 4 minutes, rotating halfway through.
- Transfer half of the beef to a tray, add another 1/2 tbsp of oil to a oven, and repeat the process with the remaining beef.
- Add 1 tbsp. oil to the now-empty cooker, then add the onions, carrots, and celery and cook for 3 minutes before adding the garlic and cooking for another minute.
- Season with salt and pepper and add the broth, onions, browned beef, basil, oregano, and thyme. Bring to the boils, then reduce to a low heat, cover, and cook for 30 minutes, stirring once or twice.
- Continue to cook, wrapped, for another 20 minutes (you can also add green beans with potatoes if you like them very soft).
- Stir in the green beans and continue to cook for another 15 minutes, or until all of the vegetables and beef are tender.
- Pour in the corn and peas and cook for 5 minutes, or until well cooked. Serve wet, garnished with parsley.
- Cooking Classy is the basis of this recipe.

130.   Pork Fillet with Green Vegetable Salad

Preparation Time: 20 Mins | Cooking Time: 6 Mins | Serves: 2 People
Ingredients:
For the Pork:
- 225g pork fillet, pork loin medallions or pork escallops
- Zest and juice of 1 lemon
- 1 tsp ground paprika
- 2 garlic cloves, peeled thinly sliced
- 1 tsp rapeseed or olive oil
- For the Yogurt and Mint Dressing:
- 5 tbsp. fat-free Greek yogurt
- Zest and juice of ½ lemon
- 2-3 tbsp. freshly chopped mint

For the Salad:
- 100g green beans, trimmed and blanched
- 100g Brussel sprouts, finely shredded
- 100g prepared cauliflower rice, cooked and cooled
- Juice of ½ lemon
- Freshly chopped mint, to garnish

Direction:
For the Pork:

- In a wide bowl placed pork, lemon zest, juice, paprika, garlic and oil. Cover and marinate for 20 mins, or longer if time allows.
- Take the pork from the marinade and roast in a hot frying pan on the hob. Stop cooking until the meat juices run clear. Take 1-2 mins, then slice. Slice the pork fillet 3 mins after frying.

For Dressing:
- Mix the dressing ingredients with the salad and bacon.
- Garnish the salad with the herbs and serve promptly.

131.   Mediterranean Beef Kofta

Number of servings: 8
Ingredients:
- 2 pounds 93% lean or leaner ground beef
- 2 tablespoons olive oil
- 1 cup minced onions
- 1 teaspoon salt
- 1 teaspoon ground cumin
- ½ teaspoon ground allspice
- 1 teaspoon ground coriander
- ½ teaspoon ground cinnamon
- ½ teaspoon dried mint leaves

Serving options:
- Hot cooked brown rice or quinoa
- Whole wheat pita
- Tzatziki sauce
- Hummus

Directions:
- Place beef, salt, cumin, allspice, coriander, onion, and mint leaves in a large bowl. Mix until just combined, making sure not to over mix.
- Take 8 bamboo skewers (around 8 inches each) and soak them in water for about 30 minutes before grilling.
- Make 8 equal portions of the meat mixture. Take one portion of the mixture and press it around one skewer, making sure to leave the ends of the skewers without meat on it.
- Make small dents, at every inch on the meat.
- Make the remaining skewers similarly. Place them on a baking sheet and chill for 20 – 30 minutes.
- Set up your grill and preheat it to medium heat. Place skewers on the grill and grill for about 3 – 4 minutes without turning the skewers. If you hurry in turning the skewers, the koftas tend to break. Do not cover the grill while cooking.
- Now turn the skewer and grill for 3 – 4 minutes. Cook the koftas similarly turning the skewers until evenly browned all over. The cooked koftas should show a reading of 160° F on the meat thermometer, in the meatiest part. 8. Serve with any one or more of the suggested serving options

Nutritional values per serving: Without serving options Calories – 216 | Fat – 12 g | Carbohydrate – 2 g | Fiber – 0.6 g | Protein – 26 g

132. Pork Rinds Crusted Salmon Patties | Gluten-Free | Nut-Free

Preparation Time: 15 Mins | Cook Time: 15 Mins | Total Time: 30 mins | Yield: 8
Ingredients:
Salmon Mixture:

- Canned Salmon or Tuna (around 14-16oz)
- 80g Red Bell Pepper
- 60g Onions
- 3 eggs
- 1 tsp Salt
- ½ tsp Black Pepper
- Optional: 1 tsp Paprika
- Optional: You can add other low-carb veggies to the mix too!

Oil for Frying Dredging:

- ½ – 1 cup of Crushed Pork Rinds
- Dip (Asian Style sauce)
- 1 tbsp Soy Sauce / Tamari / Coconut Aminos
- 1 packet of True Lemon or 1 tbsp lemon juice
- ½ tsp Sesame Oil
- 1 tsp of Lakanto Monkfruit Sweetener

Directions:

- Heat oil in a pan (medium heat).
- Using bones from salmon while cooking the dish.
- Mix salmon, red bell pepper, tomatoes, eggs, garlic, and black pepper. Not over-mixing can lead to a more balanced texture. Shape patties from the mixture. You will speed up cooling by storing the liquid in the fridge for 20-30 mins. Dredge salmon in pork rinds; make sure it's properly coated.
- Be sure to cook for 2-4 mins each hand. Cook in a mild to medium heat.

133. Pork Stir Fry

Prep: 25 mins Cook: 15 mins | Total: 40 mins | Servings: 6 | Yield: 6 servings
Ingredients:

- 5 tbsps. reduced-sodium soy sauce
- 2 tbsps. rice wine vinegar
- 1 tbsp. cornstarch
- 2 tbsp. sesame oil, divided
- 1 pound pork tenderloin, cut into strips
- 1 fresh red chile pepper, chopped
- 2 minced cloves garlic
- 1 onion, chopped
- 1 green chopped bell pepper
- 1 head bok choy, chopped
- 2 chopped
- crowns broccoli
- 1 tsp ground ginger

Directions:

- Mix soy sauce, vinegar, and cornstarch together.
- Heat 1 tbsp. oil in one wok with medium-high heat. Cook the tenderloin strips in hot oil for 2 to 4 mins. Return the wok to the heat.

- Preheat oil in same skillet on medium heat. Sauté red chile pepper and garlic in hot oil until they sizzle. Add onion, green pepper to the skillet; then cook and stir until onion begins to soften. Cook and stir chopped bok choy stalks into onions, then stir regularly, around 3 mins.
- Cook broccoli in bok choy mixture until slightly softened, around 2 mins. Add pork, sliced bok choy leaves, and soy sauce; fry and stir well. Add ginger to the rice, simmer until the bok choy and broccoli begins to wilt, 5 to 7 mins.

Nutrition per serving: 188 calories | carbohydrates 13g | fat 7.8g | cholesterol 42.1mg | sodium 540.8mg.

134. Grilled Lamb Chops with a Side of Chickpeas and Sautéed Spinach

Preparation time: 15 minutes | Cooking time: 25 minutes | Servings: 4
Ingredients:
For the lamb chops:

- 8 lamb chops, about 1 inch thick
- 2 tablespoonful olive oil
- 1 tablespoonful chopped fresh rosemary
- 1 tablespoonful chopped fresh thyme
- 1 teaspoonful garlic powder
- Salt and pepper, to taste

For the chickpeas:

- 1 can chickpeas (drained and rinsed)
- 2 tablespoonful olive oil
- 1/2 teaspoonful ground cumin
- 1/2 teaspoonful smoked paprika
- Salt and pepper, to taste

For the sautéed spinach:

- 1 tablespoonful olive oil
- 1 garlic clove (minced)
- 1 bunch spinach (washed and chopped)
- Salt and pepper, to taste

Directions:

- Preheat grill to medium-high heat.
- In a small bowl, mix together olive oil, rosemary, thyme, garlic powder, salt, and pepper.
- Brush lamb chops with the herb mixture and place on the grill. Cook for 4-5 minutes on each side, or until desired doneness.
- Meanwhile, in a medium-sized skillet over medium heat, heat olive oil. Add chickpeas, cumin, smoked paprika, salt, and pepper, and cook for 5-7 minutes, or until chickpeas are crispy.
- In another skillet over medium heat, heat olive oil. Add garlic and cook until fragrant, about 30 seconds. Add spinach, salt, and pepper, and cook until wilted, about 2-3 minutes.
- Serve grilled lamb chops with a side of crispy chickpeas and sautéed spinach.

Nutrition per serving: Calories: 458 kcal | Fat: 29 g | Saturated Fat: 8 g | Carbohydrates: 20 g | Fiber: 7 g | Protein: 32 g | Sodium: 210 mg

135. Balsamic Pork and Strawberry Salad

Number of servings: 2

Ingredients:

- ½ pound pork tenderloin, trimmed of fat
- 1 tablespoon Dijon mustard
- 1/8 teaspoon salt or to taste
- 2 cups torn lettuce leaves
- 1 ounce shredded Manchego cheese
- ¼ cup balsamic vinegar
- ½ tablespoon olive oil
- 1/8 teaspoon black pepper or to taste
- 1 cup quartered fresh strawberries

Directions:

- To make marinade: Combine vinegar and mustard in a bowl. Pour 1 ½ tablespoons of marinade into a bowl and keep it aside.
- Add meat into the remaining vinegar mixture. Turn the meat around in the bowl to coat it well.
- Cover the bowl and chill for 15 minutes.
- Set the temperature of the oven to 425°F and preheat the oven. Prepare a roasting pan by lining it with foil.
- Take out the meat from the marinade and place it in the roasting pan. The marinade is to be discarded.
- Place the roasting pan in the oven and roast until the internal temperature of the meat in the thickest part shows 145°F on the meat thermometer.
- Take out the roasting pan from the oven and let it rest for five minutes. Cut the meat into slices.

To make salad:

- Combine the retained marinade, salt, pepper, and oil.
- Combine strawberries and lettuce in a bowl.
- Divide the salad among two serving plates. Scatter cheese on top.
- Place meat slices on top and serve.

Nutrition per serving: Three ounces cooked pork with 1 ½ cups salad Calories: 278 | Fat: 11.7 g | Carbohydrates: 12.6 g | Fiber: 2.5 g | Protein: 28.5 g

136.   Greek Meatballs

Servings: 5

Ingredients:
Meatballs:

- 1 red onion, grated
- 500g / 1 lb. beef mince
- 200g / 6.5oz pork mince, or more beef
- 2 garlic cloves, minced
- 1 cup of / 60g panko breadcrumbs
- 1 egg
- 1/4 cup of fresh parsley, finely chopped
- 6 large mint leaves, finely chopped
- 1/2 tsp dried oregano
- 1 tbsp. extra virgin olive oil
- 3/4 tsp salt
- Black pepper

Cooking / Serving:

- 1/2 cup of flour any white
- 3 tbsp olive oil
- Finely chopped parsley optional, for garnish

- Tzatziki (Note 5) or Greek yoghurt

Directions:

- Add cabbage, tomatoes, pepperoni and mozzarella to a large bowl. Mix together for a few mins until the paste is consistent and very well mixed.
- If you want a smooth puffer, keep them in the fridge for an hour.
- Place heaped tsp on a work surface – could make about 35. Roll into balls.
- Heat the oil in a skillet with medium to high heat. Add enough oil to coat the skillet.
- You need to stir meatballs once in a while to avoid sticking. Brown the rolls and cook for 5-6 mins until browned all over. Pile them on a pan and repeat for leftover meatballs.
- Using oil spray on top of cooked vegetables then bake for 20 mins at 180C/350F. Pan-frying is the popular method and the meatballs are somewhat juicier.
- Serve as a side dish, such as pitas and tzatziki, for a platter or incorporate as a dinner plate with a salad.

137.   Spanish Meatballs in Garlic Tomato Sauce

Prep Time: 10 mins | Cook Time: 15 mins | Total Time: 25 mins | Servings: 4 Persons
Ingredients:
The Meatballs:

- ½ lb. or 250 g Ground Beef
- ½ lb. or 250 g Ground Pork
- 4 cloves garlic minced
- 1 Small Onion Finely Chopped
- 1 tbsp. Chopped Parsley
- 1 slice of bread soaked in milk
- 1 egg beaten
- 1 Cup of Breadcrumbs optional
- Salt and pepper to season

The Sauce:

- 2 Cloves Garlic Minced
- 4 Large Ripe Tomatoes Quartered
- 1 tbsp. Olive Oil
- ½ Cup of Tomato Paste
- ½ - 1 Tsp Smoked Paprika
- 2 Dried Cayenne Chilli Peppers
- ¼ Tsp Dried Thyme
- 1 tbsp. Honey
- Salt and Pepper to season

Directions:

- Add all the ingredients in one bowl and blend together until it is mixed. Cover and refrigerate for 30 mins.
- Roll meatballs in to golf ball size or smaller, and roll them in breadcrumbs.
- Heat some olive oil in a skillet pan, then add the meatballs and brown on all sides. You need to do this in batches. Space the meatballs out equally in the skillet.
- When done, transfer to a plate with kitchen paper and set aside.
- Mince the garlic and add it to the olive oil in a saucepan. Cook the garlic until it softens. Cook the tomatoes until soft. Blend the mixture with a blender and add remaining

ingredients. Taste the sauce and add a little more sugar, salt, or pepper.

- Move the meatballs to the saucepan and boil gently for 10 mins, then serve with fresh bread, spaghetti, rice or simply serve with toothpicks if for a crowd.

138. Lamb and White Bean Stew

Preparation time: 15 minutes | Cooking time: 2 hours | Servings: 6
Ingredients:

- 2 lbs. lamb shoulder, cut into bite-sized pieces
- 2 tablespoonful olive oil
- 1 onion (chopped)
- 2 garlic cloves (minced)
- 1 carrot (chopped)
- 1 celery stalk (chopped)
- 2 cups chicken or vegetable broth
- 1 can (14 oz.) diced tomatoes
- 1 can (15 oz.) cannellini beans, drained and rinsed
- 1/2 teaspoonful dried thyme
- 1/2 teaspoonful dried rosemary
- Salt and pepper, to taste
- Fresh parsley, chopped (for serving)

Directions:

- Heat the olive oil in a large pot or Dutch oven over medium high heat.
- Add the lamb pieces and brown on all sides, about 5-7 minutes.
- Remove the lamb from the pot and set aside.
- Add the onion, garlic, carrot, and celery to the pot and sauté for 5-7 minutes, until the vegetables are softened.
- Add the lamb back to the pot, along with the chicken or vegetable broth, diced tomatoes, cannellini beans, dried thyme, and dried rosemary.
- Bring the mixture to a boil, then reduce the heat to low and let simmer for 1.5-2 hours, stirring occasionally.
- Season with salt and pepper to taste.
- Serve hot, garnished with chopped fresh parsley.

Nutrition per serving: Calories: 380 kcal| Fat: 17 g| Carbohydrates: 27 g| Protein: 30 g| Fiber: 9 g| Sodium: 617 mg

139. Italian Shredded Pork Stew

Preparation time: 20 min | Cook: 8 hours | Makes: 9 servings (3-1/2 quarts)
Ingredients:

- 2 medium sweet potatoes, peeled and cubed
- 2 cups of chopped fresh kale
- 1 large onion, chopped
- 3 garlic cloves, minced
- 1 boneless pork shoulder butt roast
- 1 can (14 ounces) cannellini beans, rinsed and drained
- 1-1/2 tsp Italian seasoning
- ½ tsp salt
- ½ tsp pepper
- 3 cans (14-1/2 ounces each) chicken broth
- Sour cream, optional

Directions:

- Put sweet potatoes, broccoli, onion and garlic in a 5-qt. slow cooker. Place roast on vegetables. Add the ingredients. Drench soup. Cook covered over low until beef is tender.
- Cold meat mildly. Skim off the fat. Cook pork with 2 forks and return to slow cooker. If needed, use sour cream.

Nutrition info 1-1/2 cups of: 283 calories | 13g fat | 78mg cholesterol | 860mg sodium | 15g carbohydrate | 24g protein

140. Greek Turkey Meatball Gyro with Tzatziki

Number of servings: 8
Ingredients:
For meatballs:

- 2 pounds ground turkey
- 4 cloves garlic, minced
- 2 cups minced, fresh spinach
- 4 tablespoons olive oil
- ½ cup diced red onion
- 2 teaspoons oregano
- Salt to taste
- Pepper to taste

For tzatziki sauce:

- 1 cup plain Greek yogurt
- 4 tablespoons lemon juice
- 1 teaspoon garlic powder
- ½ cup grated cucumber
- 1 teaspoon dried dill
- Salt to taste

To serve:

- 1 cup thinly sliced red onion
- 2 cups diced cucumber
- 2 cups diced tomatoes
- 8 whole-wheat flatbreads

Directions:

- Combine turkey, garlic, onion, spinach, salt, and pepper in a bowl, using your hands. Make sure that you do not overmix. Divide the mixture into 24 equal portions and shape into balls.
- Pour ½ the oil into a skillet and heat over medium-high flame. Add half the meatballs and cook until brown all over. The internal temperature of the meatball should show 165° F. Transfer the meatballs onto a plate. Cook the remaining meatballs with the remaining oil. Let the meatballs sit for 15 minutes.
- To make tzatziki sauce: Combine Greek yogurt, lemon juice, garlic powder, cucumber, dill, and salt in a bowl. 4. To make gyros: Place 3 meatballs on each flatbread. Scatter ¼ cup cucumber and ¼ cup tomatoes on each flatbread. Scatter ¼ cup red onions on each. Drizzle tzatziki sauce on top and serve.

Nutrition per serving: 1 flatbread with 3 meatballs Calories – 429| Fat – 19 g| Carbohydrate – 38 g| Fiber – 19 g| Protein – 28 g

141. Grilled Pork Chops with Roasted Sweet Potatoes and Green Beans

Preparation Time: 10 minutes | Cooking Time: 30 minutes | Servings: 4

Ingredients:

For the Pork Chops:

- 4 bone-in pork chops (1-inch thick)
- 2 tablespoonful olive oil
- 1 teaspoonful dried oregano
- 1 teaspoonful garlic powder
- Salt and black pepper to taste

For the Roasted Sweet Potatoes:

- 2 medium sweet potatoes, peeled and cut into 1-inch cubes
- 1 tablespoonful olive oil
- 1 teaspoonful smoked paprika
- Salt and black pepper to taste

For the Green Beans:

- 1 pound fresh green beans, trimmed
- 2 tablespoonful olive oil
- 1 teaspoonful dried thyme
- Salt and black pepper to taste

Directions:

- Preheat the oven to 400°F (200°C).
- In a small bowl, mix together the olive oil, oregano, garlic powder, salt, and black pepper to make a marinade. Rub the pork chops all over with the marinade and set aside.
- Toss the sweet potatoes with the olive oil, smoked paprika, salt, and black pepper. Spread the sweet potatoes in a single layer on a baking sheet and roast for 20-25 minutes, or until tender and golden brown.
- In a separate bowl, toss the green beans with the olive oil, thyme, salt, and black pepper. Spread the green beans in a single layer on another baking sheet and roast for 10-15 minutes, or until tender and slightly browned.
- Preheat a grill or grill pan to medium-high heat. Grill the pork chops for 4-5 minutes per side, or until cooked through and nicely charred.
- Serve the grilled pork chops with the roasted sweet potatoes and green beans on the side.

Nutrition per serving: Calories: 450kcal | Protein: 30g | Fat: 22g | Carbohydrates: 33g | Fiber: 7g | Sugar: 8g | Sodium: 225 mg

142. Lamb Stir Fry with Green Beans

Preparation Time: 10 mins | Cook Time: 10 mins | Total Time: 20 mins | Servings: 4

Ingredients:

- 1 tsp Sichuan peppercorns
- 1 tbsp. canola oil
- 4 cloves garlic thinly sliced
- 1 pound ground American Lamb
- 1 jalapeno (thinly sliced)
- 2 tbsps. cumin
- ⅔ pound green beans (trimmed (a few large handfuls))
- 2 tbsps. soy sauce
- 2 tbsps. lime juice
- 1 tsp brown sugar
- ½ cup of cilantro coarsely chopped
- 2 green onions (thinly sliced)
- Lime wedges (for serving)
- Salt and pepper (as need)

Directions:

- Toast the peppercorns with medium heat until fragrant, about 30 seconds; let cool. To a mortar or a spice grinder, ground the peppercorns. Eject.
- Heat oil in a large cast-iron skillet or wok. Add garlic and cook, stirring for about 30 seconds. Add salt, vinegar, beef, jalapeno, cumin and Sichuan peppercorns. Cook, breaking up with a spoon and pushing tightly, about 8-10 mins.
- Meanwhile, boil beans for 45 seconds, then drain and set aside.
- In a small bowl mix soy sauce, lime juice, and brown sugar. Stir before sugar dissolves.
- Combine fried beef, green beans, soy mixture, cilantro, and green onions to combine.
- Serve over potatoes. Garnish with lime wedges on the foot.

143. Lamb, Kale, and Pomegranate Salad

Cook Time: 25 Mins | Total Time: 45 Mins

Ingredients:

- Marinade 1 1/2 cups of pomegranate juice
- 3 tbsps. extra-virgin olive oil
- 3 cloves garlic chopped
- 1 tbsp. ground ginger
- 1 tbsp. organic Ceylon cinnamon
- 2 tsp cumin
- 1 tsp unrefined sea salt
- 1/2 tsp freshly ground black pepper
- 1 4-lb leg of lamb, deboned, butterflied, and trimmed of visible fat Dressing
- 2 tsp Dijon mustard
- 2 tbsps. pomegranate balsamic vinegar
- 1/4 cup of extra-virgin olive oil Salad 5 cups of baby kale
- 2 bulbs fennel thinly sliced
- 1/2 cup of pomegranate seeds or sliced red grapes 4 cups of blanched green beans
- 2 tbsps. crumbled gorgonzola cheese
- 1/4 cup of walnut halves toasted

Directions:

- In the large resealable plastic bag, combine the marinade ingredients. Refrigerate for 8 hours or overnight after adding the lamb.
- Remove a lamb from the marinade, pat it dry, and place it on a serving platter. Turn all burners on high on the gas grill, shut the cover, and cook until hot, about 15 minutes. Clean the grates with a scraper and a brush of oil.
- Grill the lamb over medium-high heat, fat-side down, for 25–35 minutes total, depending on desired doneness, flipping halfway through. For medium-rare, aim for the internal temperature of 145°F, and for medium, aim for a temperature of 160°F. Remove a pan from the grill and cover it loosely with foil. Allow to rest for 15 minutes

before slicing thinly. Prepare the salad while you're waiting.

- Whisk together all of a dressing ingredients in a large mixing basin. Add salt and pepper to taste. Toss in the kale, fennel, pomegranate seeds, or grapes to coat. Dress salad and serve with sliced lamb, green beans, gorgonzola cheese, and toasted walnuts on a tray

144. Stuffed Eggplants

Preparation time: 30min | Cooking time: 1.2h | Servings: 4
Ingredients:

- 2 large (about 350g each) eggplants
- 1 tbsp. olive oil
- 1 onion, chopped
- 2 garlic cloves, crushed
- 2 tsp Moroccan seasoning
- 300g Coles lamb mince
- 1/2 cup basmati rice
- 3/4 cup Coles Brand Italian tomato passata
- 1/2 cup beef stock
- 100g feta, crumbled
- Spray olive oil
- 2 tbsps. Coriander leaves

Directions:

- Preheat oven to 200°C or 180°C fan. Halve eggplants lengthways. Cut a 1cm-wide border around the edge of each eggplant half. Score within the border in a diamond pattern. Use a melon baller or teaspoon to scoop out the flesh. Chop.
- Heat oil in a large deep frying pan over medium-high heat. Cook onion for 5 mins or until soft. Add the garlic and Moroccan seasoning. Cook, stirring, for 30 secs. Add the chopped eggplant. Cook for 5 mins or until soft. Add mince. Cook, stirring with a wooden spoon to break up any lumps, for 5. Stir in rice, passata and stock. Season.
- Place the eggplant shells on a lightly greased oven tray, and fill with the mince mixture. Cover with foil and bake for 45 mins. Uncover, sprinkle with feta and spray with olive oil. Cook for a further 15 mins or until the eggplant is tender and the top is golden. Top with coriander.

Nutrition per calories: calories 418kcal|protein 24g|carbs 34g|fat 21g|fiber7 g

145. Lemon Lamb Soup

Preparation time: 15min | Cooking time: 40min | Servings: 11

Ingredients:

- 5 large shoulder lamb chops, with bone in
- 12 cups water
- 1 fennel bulb, chopped 1/2 inch pieces
- 5 potatoes, chopped 1/2 inc cubes
- 1 whole lemon
- ½ - ¾ cup fresh curly-leaf parsley, chopped
- 1 -2 tablespoon salt, to taste

Directions:

- Add water and salt and bring to boil.
- Add Lamb to boiling water. 30 minutes (you can debone the meat and cut to cubes first but add bones in water with the meat cubes I prefer to cube the meat after its boiled).
- Remove the meat and/or bones and the goop on top of boiling water.
- Add the chopped fennel and boil for 5 minutes Med/high heat. -add the potatoes and boil for 10 minutes.
- Re introduce the meat if you have not cubed it first and boil 5 minutes.
- Add the parsley and boil for 5 minutes.
- Squeeze the juice of the lemon into the soup watching for the seeds and boil for another 10 minutes.

Nutrition per serving: calories 92kcal |protein 3g |carbs 21g| fat 4g | fiber 1g

146. Beef and Mushroom Barley Stew

Preparation Time: 20 minutes| Cooking Time: 2 hours | Servings: 6

Ingredients:

- 1 pound beef stew meat (cut into small pieces)
- 1 onion (diced)
- 2 cloves garlic (minced)
- 2 cups sliced mushrooms
- 2 cups low-sodium beef broth
- 1 cup water
- 1/2 cup pearl barley
- 1 teaspoonful dried thyme
- 1 teaspoonful dried rosemary
- 1 bay leaf
- 2 cups chopped kale
- Salt and freshly ground black pepper, to taste
- 1 tablespoonful olive oil

Directions:

- In a large pot, heat the olive oil over medium heat. Add the beef and sauté until browned on all sides, about 5-7 minutes.
- Add the onion and garlic to the pot and sauté until the onion is translucent, about 2-3 minutes.
- Add the sliced mushrooms to the pot and sauté until they release their liquid and start to brown, about 5-7 minutes.
- Pour in the beef broth and water, and add the pearl barley, thyme, rosemary, and bay leaf. Bring the stew to a boil, then reduce the heat to low and let it simmer for

1 1/2-2 hours, stirring occasionally, until the beef is tender and the barley is cooked.

- Add the chopped kale to the pot and cook for another 5-7 minutes until the kale is wilted.
- Season the stew with salt and freshly ground black pepper to taste. Ladle the stew into bowls and serve hot.

Nutrition per serving: Calories: 235| Fat: 8g| Carbohydrates: 19g| Protein: 22g| Fiber: 4g

147. Skillet Beef Pot Pie with Buttermilk Biscuits

Number of servings: 2

Ingredients:

- ½ tablespoon extra-virgin olive oil
- 2 cloves garlic, minced
- Salt to taste
- 6.5 ounces frozen peas
- ½ cup +1 ½ tablespoons white whole-wheat flour, divided
- ¼ cup chopped parsley + extra to garnish
- 2 tablespoons unsalted butter, cut into ¼ inch pieces
- ½ pound lean ground beef
- ½ tablespoon Dijon mustard
- ½ bag (from a 14 ounces bag) pearl onions
- ½ cup diced carrots
- 1 ½ cups low-sodium beef broth
- ¼ teaspoon baking powder
- ¼ cup buttermilk

Directions:

- Set the temperature of the oven to 400°F and preheat the oven.
- Pour oil into an ovenproof skillet and place it over medium-high heat.
- When oil is hot, add beef and cook until brown. As you stir, make sure to break the meat into pieces.
- Stir in garlic, salt, and mustard. Keep stirring for a minute.
- Add carrots, peas, and onions and mix well. Stir often until the mixture is thoroughly heated.
- Dust 1 ½ tablespoons flour over the mixture and mix well for about a minute.
- Stir in broth. Keep stirring until a bit thick.
- Add parsley and mix well. Turn off the heat.
- Place remaining flour in a bowl. Add baking powder and a pinch of salt and mix well.
- Scatter butter over the mixture and cut the butter into the flour until sand-like in texture.
- Add buttermilk and stir until just incorporated. Drop heaping tablespoonful of the batter (this is one biscuit) over the beef. You should be able to get six biscuits in all.
- Shift the skillet into the oven. Set the timing for about 20 minutes. Bake until golden brown on top.
- Sprinkle parsley on top and serve.

Nutrition per serving: 1 ½ cups| Calories: 420| Fat: 19.3 g |Carbohydrates: 35.8 g| Fiber: 6.7 g| Protein: 25.5 g

148. Sweet Potato Wedges

Preparation Time: 10 minutes | **Cooking Time:** 40 minutes | **Serving:** 2

Ingredients:

- ½ teaspoon salt
- ½ teaspoon smoked paprika
- 2 medium sweet potatoes
- ½ teaspoon ground cumin
- ½ tablespoon olive oil
- ½ teaspoon red chili powder
- ¼ teaspoon ground black pepper

Directions:

- Switch on the oven, then set it to 400 degrees F and let it preheat. Meanwhile, take a baking sheet, line it with a parchment sheet, and set it aside until required. Scrub the potatoes, wash them, and then cut them into wedges.
- Scatter the potato wedges on the prepared baking sheet, drizzle with oil, and sprinkle with all the seasonings, toss until coated, and then spread in a single layer. Place the prepared baking sheet into the oven and then bake for 35 to 40 minutes until nicely browned and crisp, tossing halfway.
- Meal Prep: Cool the potato wedges completely, divide them evenly between two meal prep containers, and then store them in the refrigerator for up to 3 days or freeze for up to 1 month. When ready to eat, bring the potato wedges to room temperature, microwave for 2 to 3 minutes until hot, and then serve with tahini sauce.

Nutrition per serving: Calories: 291 Cal | Total Fats: 11.7 g | Saturated Fat: 1.7 g | Carbohydrate: 44.4 g | Sugar: 4.1 g | Fiber: 8 g | Protein: 6 g

149. Fig and Ricotta Toast

Number of servings: 2

Ingredients:

- 2 slices crusty whole-grain bread, toasted
- 2 fresh figs or four dried figs, sliced
- 2 teaspoons honey
- ½ cup part-skim ricotta cheese
- 2 teaspoons toasted, sliced almonds
- A large pinch flaky sea salt

Directions:

- Spread four tablespoons of part-skim ricotta cheese on each toast. Place fig slices over the toast.
- Scatter almonds on the toast. Sprinkle flaky sea salt on top and serve

Nutrition per serving: One toast Calories: 252 | Fat: 9.1 g | Carbohydrates: 32.1 g | Fiber: 4.3 g | Protein: 12.5 g

150. Greek Yogurt with Mixed Berries and a Drizzle of Honey

Preparation time: 5 minutes | **cooking time:** 0 minutes | **Servings:** 2

Ingredients:

- 1 cup Greek yogurt
- 1 cup mixed berries (such as strawberries, blueberries, and raspberries)
- 2 tablespoons honey

Directions:

- In a bowl, mix together the Greek yogurt and honey until well combined. Wash the mixed berries and pat them dry with a paper towel.
- Divide the yogurt mixture evenly between two bowls. Top the yogurt with the mixed berries. Drizzle honey over the berries.

Nutrition per serving: Calories: 195 | Fat: 2g | Carbohydrates: 36g | Protein: 11g | Fiber: 3g | Sugar: 30g

151. Pumpkin Banana Oats Breakfast Cookies

Number of servings: 24

Ingredients:

- 4 cup dry oats or your choice
- 2 ripe bananas, mashed
- ½ cup natural applesauce
- 6 tablespoons hemp hearts
- ½ teaspoon salt
- 2/3 cup pure pumpkin puree
- 2/3 cup pure maple syrup
- 2 teaspoons vanilla extract
- 2 teaspoons ground cinnamon
- 1 teaspoon baking powder

Directions:

- Prepare 2 baking sheets by greasing with cooking spray.
- Add 3 cups of oats into the food processor bowl and give short pulses until most of it is ground.
- Combine mashed banana, pumpkin puree, apple sauce, maple syrup, and vanilla in a mixing bowl and whisk until smooth.
- Stir in the ground oats, 1 cup oats, cinnamon, baking powder, hemp hearts, and salt. Mix until just incorporated, making sure not to over-mix.
- Scoop the batter onto the baking sheet. Leave a sufficient gap between the cookies. Press the cookies to flatten, using a fork.
- Bake them in batches. Set up the temperature of your oven to 350° F and preheat the oven. Place a baking sheet in the oven and set the timer for 12 minutes. When the cookies are baked, you can see a light brown color on the bottom of the cookies.
- Cool for a few minutes on the baking sheet. Transfer the cookies onto a cooling rack. Cool completely.
- Transfer the cookies into an airtight container. Store the cookies at room temperature. It can last for 6 – 7 days.

Nutrition per serving: Calories – 104 | Fat – 2 g | Carbohydrate – 20 g | Fiber – 2 g | Protein – 3 g

152. Energy Bar

Number of servings: 16

Ingredients:

- 2 cups roughly chopped almonds
- 1 cup honey or maple syrup
- 4 tablespoons melted coconut oil
- 3 cups uncooked oats
- 2 cups almond butter or peanut butter
- 1 teaspoon salt (optional)
- 2 cups dried cranberries or chocolate chips or dried tart cherries or dried fruit or nuts

Directions:

- Combine oats, almonds, and cranberries in a large bowl.
- Combine coconut oil and almond butter in a small saucepan. Place the saucepan over low heat and cook the mixture until smooth.
- Turn off the heat. Add honey and stir. Pour into the bowl of oat mixture and mix well.
- Spread the mixture into a large baking dish. Press the mixture well onto the bottom of the dish.
- Make marking for 16 equal size bars. Keep the dish covered in cling wrap and chill for 3-8 hours.
- Now cut over the markings. Place in an airtight container in the refrigerator. It can last for 6-7 days in the refrigerator or for a month in the freezer. Thaw before serving.

Nutrition per serving: Calories: 412| Fat: 26 g| Carbohydrates: 36 g| Fiber: 7 g| Protein: 12 g

153. Hummus Bell Pepper and Feta Crackers

Number of servings: 2
Ingredients:

- 4 tablespoons hummus
- ¼ cup crumbled feta cheese
- 2 large whole-grain crispbread like Wasa sourdough whole-grain crispbread
- ¼ cup diced bell peppers

Directions:

- Spread two tablespoons of hummus on each crispbread. Scatter feta cheese and bell pepper on top and serve

Nutrition per serving: Calories: 136| Fat: 1.7 g | Carbohydrates: 13.1 g| Fiber: 3.6 g| Protein: 6 g

154. Mango and Strawberry Smoothie

Preparation Time: 5 minutes | Cooking Time: 0 minutes|
Serving: 1
Ingredients:

- ½ of a frozen banana, peeled
- ¼ teaspoon ground turmeric
- ¼ cup frozen strawberries
- ¼ teaspoon ginger powder
- ¼ cup frozen mango pieces
- ¼ cup Greek yogurt
- 1 tablespoon honey
- ¼ cup almond milk, unsweetened

Directions:

- Take an 8-ounce mason jar, and place banana, berries, mango, turmeric, ginger and honey in it. Seal the mason jar with its lid and store it in the refrigerator for 3 days.
- When ready to drink, add yogurt and milk into the mason jar and then pulse with an immersion blender until smooth. Serve straight away.

Nutrition per serving: Calories: 156 Cal| Total Fats: 1 g| Saturated Fat: 0.4 g| Carbohydrate: 33 g| Sugar: 3 g| Fiber: 3 g| Protein: 7 g

CHAPTER 10: PIZZA, WRAPS AND SANDWICHES

155. Hot Sandwiches with Cheese, Tomatoes and Greens

Preparation Time: 5 minutes | Serves: 4
Ingredients:
- 4 White bread
- 1 Green onion, bundle
- 1 Tomato
- 4 tbsp White cheese
- 2 tsp Butter
- 1 Parsley, bundle

Directions:
- Dry the slices of bread. Chop green onions and parsley. Cheese mixed with butter, onions, and herbs. Put the finished curd on the bread. Put thin slices of tomato on top.
- Bake sandwiches in the microwave at full power for 2–3 minutes.

Nutrition per serving: Calories: 182 Kcal Fat: 7.1 g. | Protein: 6.6 g. | Carbs: 22.3 g

156. Spanakopita

Number of servings: 12
Ingredients:
- 2 pounds frozen spinach, thawed
- 3 cups crumbled, full-fat feta cheese
- 2 tablespoons finely chopped fresh dill
- 17 sheets frozen, whole-wheat phyllo dough, thawed
- 2 large leeks, white and light green parts, thinly sliced
- 4 large eggs, beaten
- 1 teaspoon sea salt
- 4 tablespoons olive oil, to brush
- 1 teaspoon pepper

Directions:
- Squeeze out as much moisture from the spinach as possible.
- Place spinach in a bowl along with feta, leeks, salt, pepper, dill, and eggs. Mix well.
- Take 2 pie plates of 9 inches each and line each with a sheet of phyllo dough. Brush oil over the sheets.
- Place one more sheet in each pan, slightly away from the middle of the pie pan. The sheet should overhang by around 2 inches. Brush oil once again.
- Repeat the previous step 4 more times, but change the placing of the sheet from another point. For this, you can rotate the pie pans a little and then place the sheet. So you should have overhanging dough all around the pie pans. Make sure to now press the dough layers onto the bottom of the pans.
- Divide the spinach mixture among the pie pans. Gently lift the overhanging dough portions and place over the filling.
- Tear the remaining dough sheets into 2 halves and place them on the top of the dough. Crimp the edges to seal. Brush some oil on top.

- Set up the temperature of your oven to 375° F and preheat the oven. Bake the pies until golden brown. Cut each pie into 6 slices and serve

Nutrition per serving: Calories – 286| Fat – 15 g| Carbohydrate – 26 g| Fiber – 4 g| Protein – 13 g

157. Crockpot Chicken Tacos

Prep Time: 5 minutes | Cook Time: 8 hours | Total Time: 8 hours 5 minutes
Ingredients:
- 4 large boneless skinless chicken breasts
- 1 packet Taco Seasoning or 3 Tbsp Homemade Taco Seasoning
- 2 cups of pico de gallo or 1 can diced tomatoes and chiles
- Corn or flour tortillas
- Favorite Toppings: Cheese lettuce, tomatoes, onions, cilantro, sour cream, salsa, sliced avocados, or guacamole

Directions
- In the crockpot, place the boneless, skinless chicken breasts.
- Season with taco seasoning and serve.
- Toss in the pico de gallo or canned tomatoes and chilies (liquid and all)
- Cook the chicken on low heat for 6 to 8 hours.
- Pull a chicken breast apart with two forks to shred the chicken. Allow for 30 minutes in the crockpot.
- Fill the tortillas with shredded chicken.
- Cheese, lettuce, tomatoes, onion, cilantro, sour cream, avocados, and other toppings can be added.

Nutrition Per Serving: Calories: 197kcal | Carbohydrates: 26g | Protein: 18g | Fat: 3g | Cholesterol: 48mg | Sodium: 648mg | Potassium: 343mg | Fiber: 2g | Sugar: 7g

158. Chicken Lettuce Wraps

Preparation Time: 10 minutes | Cooking Time: 20 minutes | Serving: 3
Ingredients:
- 10 ounces' chicken thighs, boneless, skinless, cut into bite-sized pieces
- ½ teaspoon minced garlic
- 1 teaspoon coriander
- 1 teaspoon crushed red pepper
- 1 tablespoon olive oil
- 1 teaspoon dried rosemary
- 1 zucchini, cut in circles
- 1 teaspoon dried mint

To Assemble:
- 3 big leaves of lettuce
- 3 tablespoons hummus
- 3 tablespoons cashew sauce

Directions:
- Take a skillet pan, place it over medium heat, add oil, and when hot, add chicken pieces, and then cook until no longer pink.
- Switch heat to medium-high level, stir in coriander, garlic, mint, rosemary, and red pepper and then continue cooking for 10 to 15 minutes until almost cooked. Add

zucchini, stir until mixed and continue cooking for 4 minutes or until cooked.

- Meal Prep: Let the chicken and zucchini cool completely, then divide it evenly among three meal prep containers and cover it with a lid. Store the containers in the refrigerator for up to 5 days or freeze for up to 1 month.
- When ready to eat, thaw the container overnight in the refrigerator, and microwave for 2 to 3 minutes. Assemble the wrap and for this, take a lettuce leaf, spread hummus on it, top with chicken and zucchini, drizzle with cashew sauce, wrap it and then serve.

Nutrition per serving: Calories: 397 Cal| Total Fats: 23 g| Saturated Fat: 4 g| Carbohydrate: 34 g| Sugar: 9 g| Fiber: 10 g| Protein: 20 g

159. Oatmeal Pancakes

Preparation Time: 10 minutes | Cooking Time: 10 minutes| Serving: 2
Ingredients:
- 1/2 cup oats
- 1/8 teaspoon baking soda
- 1 egg
- 1 teaspoon vanilla extract, unsweetened
- 2 ½ tablespoons yogurt
- 1 tablespoon honey
- 1 teaspoon coconut oil

Directions:
- Plug in a food processor, add oats in it, and then pulse until ground. Take a medium bowl, crack the egg in it, add vanilla, honey and yogurt and whisk until combined. Add oats and baking soda and then stir until incorporated. Take a skillet pan, place it over medium-low heat, add oil and when it melts, ladle some batter in it.
- Shape the batter like a pancake and then cook for 3 to 4 minutes per side until firm and golden brown. Repeat with the remaining batter and prepare more pancakes.
- Meal Prep: Let the pancakes cool completely, then divide them evenly between two meal prep containers and cover them with a lid. Store the container in the refrigerator for up to 5 days or freeze for up to 1 month.
- When ready to eat, thaw the container overnight in the refrigerator, microwave for 2 to 3 minutes until hot, and then serve.

Nutrition per serving: Calories: 233 Cal |Total Fats: 12 g |Saturated Fat: 7 g| Carbohydrate: 24 g| Sugar: 10 g| Fiber: 2 g| Protein: 7 g

160. Canapes with Cheese, Tomato, and Salmon

Cook time: 30 minutes | Serves: 4
Ingredients:
- 3 Tomato
- 5 Bread, piece
- 10 Salmon, slices
- 4 oz Cheese
- 2 oz Butter

Directions:

- Bread cut into slices and dry on the baking sheet. Cut the cheese into thin triangles, cut the salmon into thin slices, and cut the tomatoes into very thin slices.
- Spread the dried bread with softened butter, lay a triangle of cheese and a slice of tomato on each piece, and folded salmon slices in half on top.
- Place the canapes on baking paper and bake in a preheated oven to 350 degrees for 15 minutes, until the cheese becomes sticky. Serve hot.

Nutrition per serving: Calories: 252 Kcal| Fat: 16.7 g. | Protein: 9.5 g. | Carbs: 16.3 g

161. Simple Raw Tomato Juice

Ingredients:
- 1 large tomato
- 1 tbsp Honey or maple syrup, as need Ice

Direction:
- Get wedges out of your tomato.
- In a mixer, mix the tomato slice, sugar, and ice.
- Blend for a few minutes on strong (until well blended).

Nutrition per serving: Calories: 149| total Fat: 0g| Cholesterol: 0mg| sodium: 13mg| carbohydrates: 38g| fiber: 2g

162. Pita Pizza

Number of servings: 4
Ingredients:
- 8 slices bacon
- 4 tablespoons extra-virgin olive oil
- 4 tablespoons pesto
- ● 1 tomato, chopped
- ● 1 cup chopped spinach
- ● ½ onion, chopped
- ● ½ cup
- ● ½ cup chopped fresh mushrooms
- ● 2 avocados, peeled, pitted, chopped
- ● 4 eggs, beaten
- ● 4 whole-wheat pita bread rounds
- ● Salt to taste
- ● 1 cup shredded cheddar cheese
- ● Pepper to taste

Directions:
- Place a skillet over medium-high flame. Add bacon and cook until brown. Stir occasionally.
- Remove bacon with a slotted spoon and place on a plate lined with paper towels.
- Add onions into the skillet and cook until onions turn pink. Transfer the onion into a bowl.
- To make scrambled eggs: Pour oil into the skillet. When the oil is heated, add eggs into the pan and cook until the eggs are cooked. Stir often until the eggs are cooked. Turn off the heat.
- Set up the temperature of your oven to 350° F and preheat the oven. Prepare a large baking sheet by lining it with parchment paper.
- Place the pita bread rounds on the prepared baking sheet. Spread a tablespoon of pesto on each. Divide equally the bacon and scrambled eggs among the pita rounds and spread over the pitas.

- Scatter tomatoes, spinach, and mushrooms. Finally, top with cheddar cheese.
- Place the baking sheet in the oven and bake for 10 minutes, until the cheese melts. 9. Garnish with avocado slices and serve.

Nutrition per serving: 1 pita pizza Calories – 873 | Fat – 62.9 g | Carbohydrate – 43.5 g | Fiber – 9.5 g | Protein – 36.8 g

163.   Shrimp, Avocado & Feta Wrap

Number of servings: 2
Ingredients:

- 6 ounces cooked, chopped shrimp
- ½ cup diced tomato
- ¼ cup crumbled feta cheese
- 2 whole wheat tortillas
- ½ cup diced avocado
- 2 scallions, sliced
- Pepper to taste
- 2 tablespoons lime juice
- Salt to taste

Directions:

- Stir together shrimp, tomatoes, lime juice, avocado, feta, and scallions in a bowl.
- Add salt and pepper to taste.
- Divide the mixture among the tortillas. Wrap and serve.

Nutrition per serving: Calories – 371 | Fat – 5.9 g | Carbohydrate – 34.3 g | Fiber – 6.4 g | Protein – 28.8 g

164.   Portobello Mushroom Pizzas with Arugula Salad

Preparation time: 30min | Cooking time: 15min | Servings: 4
Ingredients:

- 8 large portobello mushroom caps (about 4 oz. each), gills removed (see Tip)
- 2 tablespoons olive oil plus 1 tsp., divided
- ½ teaspoon ground pepper, divided
- ½ cup pizza or tomato sauce
- 2 cups lightly packed baby spinach, chopped
- ½ cup sun-dried tomatoes (about 8), chopped
- 1 (14 ounce) can artichoke hearts, rinsed and chopped
- ½ cup shredded part-skim mozzarella cheese
- ¼ cup crumbled feta cheese
- ½ teaspoon dried Italian seasoning
- 1 tablespoon lemon juice
- 2 cups lightly packed baby arugula
- ¼ cup fresh basil leaves, thinly sliced

Directions:

- Preheat oven to 400 degrees F. Line a large baking sheet with foil and set a wire rack on it. Brush tops of portobello caps with 1 Tbsp. oil and place them, undersides-up, on the rack. Roast for 10 minutes. Flip and roast for 5 minutes more.
- Remove the portobellos from the oven and carefully flip them back over so that the undersides are up. Season with 1/4 tsp. pepper. Spread 1 Tbsp. sauce inside each cap. Divide spinach, sun-dried tomatoes, artichokes, mozzarella, and feta among the caps. Sprinkle with Italian

seasoning. Return the portobellos to the oven and bake until the cheese is melted and starting to brown, 10 to 15 minutes.

- Meanwhile, whisk the remaining 1 Tbsp. plus 1 tsp. oil, the remaining 1/8 tsp. pepper, and lemon juice in a medium bowl. Add arugula and toss to coat. -Garnish the portobello pizzas with basil and serve with the arugula salad.

Nutrition per serving: calories 246kcal | protein 14g | carbs 25g | fat 4g | fiber 7g

165.   Caesar Egg Salad Lettuce Wraps – Low Carb, Gluten

Free Yield: 4 Servings
Ingredients

- 6 large hard-boiled eggs, peeled and chopped
- 3 tbsp creamy caesar dressing
- 3 tbsp mayonnaise
- ½ cup of Parmesan cheese, shredded, divided
- Cracked black pepper, as need
- 4 large romaine lettuce leaves

Direction:

- Combine diced eggs, creamy caesar sauce, mayonnaise, 1/4 cup of Parmesan cheese and crushed black pepper.
- Spoon on roman leaves and top with remaining Parmesan cheese

Nutrition per serving: Calories: 254 | Fat: 22g | Carbohydrates: 2.75g | Protein: 13.5g

CHAPTER 11: STAPLES, SOUPS, SAUCES, DIPS AND DRESSINGS

166.   Pinto Bean Dip

Total Time: 25 min| Makes: 25-30 servings
Ingredients:

- 30 ounces' pinto beans, rinsed and drained
- 1-1/4 tsp salt, divided
- ¼ tsp pepper
- 1/8 to ¼ tsp hot pepper sauce
- 3 ripe avocados, peeled and pitted
- 4 tsp lemon juice
- 1 cup of sour cream
- ½ cup of mayonnaise
- 1 envelope taco seasoning
- 1 cup of sliced green onions
- 2 medium tomatoes, chopped
- 1-1/2 cups of shredded cheddar cheese
- 2-1/4 ounces sliced ripe olives, drained
- Tortilla chips

Directions:

- Cut beans with a fork and stir in ¾ tsp salt, pepper and pepper sauce. Stretched onto a 12-in. plate.
- Mash avocados and lemon juice; scatter over bean mixture. Put the sour cream, mayonnaise and taco seasoning over the avocado.
- Add tomatoes, mushrooms, cheese and olives. Serve with chips.

167.   Minestrone Soup

Total time: 45 min | Yield: 6 servings
Ingredients:

- 2 tbsp. extra-virgin olive oil
- 1 large onion, diced
- 4 minced cloves garlic
- 2 stalks diced celery
- 1 large diced carrot
- 1/3 pound green beans, trimmed and cut into ½-inch pieces (about 1 ½ cups of)
- 1 tsp dried oregano
- 1 tsp dried basil
- Kosher salt and freshly ground pepper
- 1 28-ounce can no-salt-added diced tomatoes
- 1 14-ounce can crushed tomatoes
- 6 cups of low sodium chicken broth
- 1 15-ounce can low sodium kidney beans, drained and rinsed
- 1 cup of elbow pasta
- 1/3 cup of grated parmesan cheese
- 2 tbsp. chopped fresh basil

Directions:

- Heat oil in a big pot over medium-high heat. Cook onion until translucent, about 4 mins. Add garlic, cook 30 seconds. Add the celery and carrot and simmer until they soften, about 5 mins. Add green beans, dried oregano and basil, ¾ tsp salt and pepper as need; simmer for 3 mins. Add the diced and pounded tomatoes and chicken broth to the pot and simmer. Reduce heat to medium-low, cook 10 mins.
- Add beans and the pasta and cook until pasta and vegetables are tender, about 10 mins. Salt season. Ladle in bowls and cover with parmesan basil.

168.   Healthy Mediterranean 7-Layer Dip Recipe

Preparation Time: 15 minutes | Total Time: 15 minutes
Ingredients:

- 8 oz. hummus I prefer Sabra
- 1 tomato diced
- 1/2 cup of diced cucumber
- 1/2 cup of nonfat Greek yogurt
- 1/8 tsp salt
- 1/4 tsp paprika
- 2 canned artichoke heart chopped
- 2 roasted red peppers 4 halves, diced
- 1/4 cup of crumbled feta cheese
- 2 tbsp minced flat-leaf parsley
- Kalamata olives chopped (optional), for garnish

Dedication:

- Spread the hummus equally on the bottom of an 8" by 8" square serving plate. Overtop, layer the tomatoes and cucumber.
- Using a rubber spatula, carefully spread the yogurt over the veggies. Season the yogurt with salt and paprika before serving.
- Layer an artichoke heart, roasted red peppers, and feta cheese on top of the yogurt. Sprinkle a parsley on top and serve with olives as a garnish.
- Serve with fresh veggies, pita chips, or crackers to round off the meal.

169.   Zucchini-Basil Soup

Preparation time: 15min | Cooking time: 30min | Servings: 5
Ingredients:

- 2 pounds' zucchini, trimmed and cut crosswise into thirds
- 3/4 cup chopped onion
- 2 garlic cloves, chopped
- 1/4 cup olive oil
- 4 cups water, divided
- 1/3 cup packed basil leaves

Directions:

- Julienne skin (only) from half of zucchini with slicer; toss with 1/2 teaspoon salt and drain in a sieve until wilted, at least 20 minutes. Coarsely chop remaining zucchini.
- Cook onion and garlic in oil in a 3- to 4- quarts heavy saucepan over medium-low heat, stirring occasionally, until softened, about 5 minutes. Add chopped zucchini and 1 teaspoon salt and cook, stirring occasionally, 5 minutes. Add 3 cups water and simmer, partially covered, until tender, about 15 minutes. Purée soup with basil in 2 batches in a blender (use caution when blending hot liquids).

- Bring remaining cup water to a boil in a small saucepan and blanch julienned zucchini 1 minute. Drain in a sieve set over a bowl (use liquid to thin soup if necessary).
- Season soup with salt and pepper. Serve in shallow bowls with julienned zucchini mounded on top.

Nutrition per serving: calories 200kcal | carbs 18g

170. Skillet Chicken with Garlic Herb Butter Sauce

Preparation time: 8min | Cooking time: 15min | Servings: 4
Ingredients:

- 4 (6 oz) boneless, skinless chicken breasts
- 1 1/2 Tbsp minced garlic (4 cloves)
- 1 Tbsp olive oil
- Salt and freshly ground black pepper
- 1/3 cup low-sodium chicken stock or dry white wine
- 4 Tbsp. unsalted butter, divided
- 2 tsp chopped fresh sage*
- 1 tsp chopped fresh thyme
- 1 tsp chopped fresh rosemary

Directions:

- Heat a large 12-inch skillet over medium high heat. Pound thicker parts of chicken with the flat side of a meat mallet to even their thickness.
- Dab chicken dry with paper towels, then season both sides of chicken with salt and pepper. Add oil to skillet, then add chicken.
- Cook chicken about 5 - 6 minutes per side or until center registers 165 degrees on an instant read thermometer. Transfer to a plate.
- Reduce burner temperature slightly, then melt 1 1/2 Tbsp. butter in same skillet. Add in garlic and sage and sauté until garlic is golden brown, about 30 seconds.
- Pour in chicken broth and scrape up browned bits from bottom of pan. Dice remaining butter into 3 pieces then add to skillet along with thyme and rosemary. Stir until butter is melted.
- Return chicken to pan and spoon sauce over top. Serve warm.

Nutrition per serving: calories 335kcal | protein 36g | carbs 1g | fat 19g

171. Guacamole

Preparation time: 45 minutes | Serves: 10
Ingredients:

- 1 Avocado
- 3 Green chili pepper
- 1 Bell green pepper
- 1/2 Onion
- 1/2 Tomato
- 1/2 tsp Lemon juice
- 4 Coriander Seeds Salt, to taste

Directions:

- Finely chop the onion, green pepper, and tomato. Coriander seeds are crushed in a mortar or directly on the cutting board with the flat side of a knife. Divide the avocado in two, remove the bone.
- Spoon pick the flesh from the rind and put in a bowl. Fork crumble the pulp. Add onion, pepper, chili, tomato

and coriander, salt and mix the lemon juice so that the vegetables do not lose color. Mix everything well, put in a serving cup. Cover with foil and refrigerate.
- Remove the chili peppers before serving. This hot sauce is great for cold meats or as an appetizer with crackers.

Nutritional per serving (1 tbsp.): Calories: 13 Kcal | Fat: 1.1 g. | Protein: 0.3 g. | Carbs: 1 g

172. Panna Cotta with Berry Sauce

Preparation Time: 4 hours 5 mins | Cook Time: 15 mins | Total Time: 4 hours 20 mins | Servings: 6 dessert cups of Ingredients
Ingredients for Panna Cotta:

- 1 cup of whole milk
- 2 ½ tsp unflavored gelatin
- 2 cups of heavy whipping cream
- ½ cup of + 1 Tbsp sugar
- Pinch salt
- 1 tsp vanilla extract
- 1 cup of sour cream

Ingredients for Berry Sauce:

- 2 cups of berries divided
- 3 Tbsp granulated sugar
- ½ Tbsp lemon juice

Dedication:
How to Make Panna Cotta:

- When the sauce is cold, sprinkle 1 cup of milk on top of the gelatin. Let stand 3-5 mins, or until softened. Switch heat up to medium/low and cook slowly for around 5 mins (do not boil).
- Add 2 cups of strong whipping cream, ½ cup of + 1 Tbsp sugar, 1 tsp vanilla and a pinch of salt. Continue swirling the mixture for another five mins to get sugar dissolved (do not boil). Let it cool off for 5 mins.
- Using a medium cup of to mix sour cream. Whisk in the warm milk. Divide it in 8 ramekins. Keep refrigerated until completely set.

How to Make Berry Sauce:

- In a shallow saucepan, mix 1 cup of fruit, ½ tbsps. lemon juice and 3 tbsps. sugar. Bring to a low boil and simmer 4-5 mins.
- Add remaining 1 cup of fresh berries and mix well. Spoon it on the warm desserts or use sweet syrup to warm the cold desserts.

Nutrition per serving:
Panna Cotta with Berry Sauce: Calories 494 | Fat 38g | Cholesterol 132mg | Sodium 82mg | Potassium 195mg | Carbohydrates 34g | Fiber 1g | Sugar 30g | Protein 5g | Calcium 144mg | Iron 0.2mg

173. Cauliflower Cream Sauce

Preparation time: 10min | Cooking time: 10min | Servings: 5
Ingredients:

- 1 head of cauliflower, roughly chopped
- 2 cups vegetable broth
- 2 cups non-dairy milk (such as soy or almond)
- 3 cloves garlic, peeled
- ¼ cup nutritional yeast
- 2 teaspoons white miso paste

- ½ teaspoon salt (or to taste)

Directions:

- Add the cauliflower, vegetable broth, nondairy milk, and garlic to a big pot, and bring to a simmer. Cook for about 10 minutes, until the cauliflower is very soft and falls apart when pierced with a fork.
- Now blend up the cauliflower mixture. You can use an emersion blender and blend everything together directly in the pot, or you can use a standing blender and blend the cauliflower and cooking liquid in batches, being careful not to fill the blender too high so the hot liquid doesn't explode out the top. Add the nutritional yeast, white miso paste, and salt and blend to combine.
- If you find your sauce is too thin, return the sauce to the pan and cook it down a bit more stirring often so it doesn't burn. If it is too thick, add a bit more vegetable broth or water.
- The ways to use this sauce are endless. Toss with pasta, mix into a casserole, top on pizza, make creamy scalloped potatoes, drizzle over baked potatoes, use in lasagna, you name it!

Nutrition per serving: calories 52kcal

174. Greek Lemon Chicken Soup

Preparation Time: 10 minutes | Cooking Time: 20 minutes | Serving: 6

Ingredients:

- 30 ounces canned cannellini beans, rinsed, drained
- 1-pound chicken thighs, boneless, skinless, cut into
- 1-inch chunks
- 1 medium white onion, peeled, diced
- 1 teaspoon salt
- 2 tablespoons lemon juice
- 3 medium carrots, peeled, diced
- 4 cups baby spinach, fresh
- ½ teaspoon ground black pepper
- 2 teaspoons minced garlic
- 2 stalks celery, diced
- ½ teaspoon dried thyme
- 2 tablespoons olive oil, divided
- 8 cups chicken stock
- 2 tablespoons chopped parsley leaves
- 2 bay leaves
- 2 tablespoons chopped dill

Directions:

- Prepare the chicken and for this, cut the chicken thighs into 1-inch pieces and then season with ½ teaspoon and ¼ teaspoon ground black pepper.
- Take a large pot, place it over medium heat, add 1 tablespoon oil and when hot, add chicken thigh pieces and then cook for 3 to 4 minutes per side until golden.
- Transfer chicken pieces to a plate, add 1 tablespoon oil into the pot, and when hot, add celery, garlic, carrot, and onion and then cook for 4 minutes until tender.
- Stir in thyme, cook for 1 minute, add bay leaves, pour in the chicken stock, and bring the soup to a boil. Then switch heat to medium-low level, add chicken pieces and cannellini beans and cook the soup for 10 to 15 minutes until soup has thickened slightly.

- Add spinach, stir until mixed and cook for 2 minutes until spinach leaves have wilted. Then stir in dill, parsley, and lemon juice, stir in remaining salt and black pepper and remove the pot from heat.
- Meal Prep: Let the soup cool completely, then divide them evenly among six meal prep containers and cover it with a lid. Store the containers in the refrigerator for up to 5 days or freeze for up to 1 month.
- When ready to eat, thaw the container overnight in the refrigerator, microwave for 2 to 3 minutes until hot, and then serve.

Nutrition per serving: Calories: 241 Cal| Total Fats: 9 g| Saturated Fat: 2 g| Carbohydrate: 18 g| Sugar: 1 g| Fiber: 4 g| Protein: 19 g

175. Homemade Mayo

Preparation time: 5 minutes | Serves: 10

Ingredients

- 7 oz Olive oil
- 1/2 cup Milk
- 1 tsp Sugar
- 1 tbsp Mustard
- 1 tbsp Lemon Juice Salt, to taste

Directions:

- Add all ingredients except lemon juice in one measuring cup. Beat the blender until a thick white mass is formed, about 3-4 minutes. Add lemon juice while continuing to beat.

Nutrition per serving (1 tbsp): Calories: 102 Kcal Fat: 12.1 g. | Protein: 0.4 g. | Carbs: 0.1 g

176. Avocado Spread

Preparation time: 5 min | Cooking time: 0 min | Servings: 1

Ingredients:

- 2 Medium Ripe Avocados
- ¼ teaspoon Salt
- Black Pepper, a generous pinch
- ½ Lemon, juice only, see note 1
- 2 tablespoons Extra Virgin Olive Oil, see note 2
- 1 tablespoon Chia Seeds, see note 3
- Chili Peppers, to taste

Directions:

- Half the avocados and remove pits. Take out the flesh and transfer it into a bowl. Mash it until smooth (or to your liking). Add salt, pepper, lemon juice, olive oil, chia seeds and stir well.
- Taste it and season, if needed. Finely chop chili and either stir it into the spread or just sprinkle some over.

Nutrition per serving: calories 60kcal |protein 1g |carbs 3g | fat 6g | fiber 2g

177. Pesto

Preparation time: 10 minutes | Serves: 10

Ingredients:

- 4 fl. oz Olive oil
- 2 oz Green basil
- 2 oz Parmesan
- 2 Garlic, clove

- 1 tsp Pine nuts Salt, to taste

Directions:

- Basil wash and dry. Cut garlic cloves into large pieces. Grate the parmesan. Mix all ingredients in a blender until smooth. Add olive oil to taste.

Nutrition per serving (1 tbsp): Calories: 81 Kcal Fat: 8.7 g. | Protein: 1.5 g. | Carbs: 0.3 g.

178. Garlic Sauce

Preparation time: 15 minutes | Serves: 10
Ingredients:

- 1 cup Chicken broth
- 1 Garlic, clove
- 1 tbsp. Wheat flour
- 1 tbsp. Vinegar
- 1 tsp Butter Salt, to taste

Directions:

- Fry the butter and flour in a pan over medium heat. Add broth. Salt, add vinegar. Smash the garlic in the mortar, add to the mixture. Boil the sauce, stirring constantly, in a small saucepan over low heat for 10 minutes. The sauce is very good for boiled meat, fish or poultry.

Nutrition per serving (1 tbsp): Calories: 9 Kcal Fat: 0.4 g. | Protein: 0.2 g. | Carbs: 0.9 g

179. Tomato Basil Soup

Preparation Time: 5 minutes | Cooking Time: 10 minutes | Serving: 1
Ingredients:

- ¼ cup chopped white onion
- 1 teaspoon minced garlic
- 14.5-ounces fire-roasted diced tomatoes
- ¼ teaspoon salt
- 1/3 cup chicken broth
- 2 large basil leaves, chopped
- 2 teaspoons olive oil

Directions:

- Take a small saucepan, place it over medium heat, add oil, and when hot, add onion and garlic and cook for 1 minute until fragrant. Add tomatoes, pour in the broth, and then simmer the soup for 5 minutes. Remove the pan from the heat and puree it using an immersion blender. Add salt and stir until mixed. Meal Prep: Let the soup cool completely, then pour it into a meal prep container and cover it with a lid.
- Store the container in the refrigerator for up to 5 days or freeze for up to 1 month. When ready to eat, thaw the container overnight in the refrigerator, microwave for 2 to 3 minutes until hot, and then serve.

Nutrition per serving: Calories: 233 Cal | Total Fats: 11.2 g | Saturated Fat: 2 g | Carbohydrate: 32.1 g | Sugar: 2.7 g | Fiber: 4.7 g | Protein: 6.3 g

CHAPTER 12: DESERTS

180.   Banana Smoothie Bowl

Preparation time: 10min | Cooking time: 0min | Servings: 1
Ingredients:

- 2 frozen bananas, peeled and sliced
- ¼ cup milk – almond, soy, etc.
- 1–2 tablespoons nut butter
- Pinch cinnamon, optional

Directions:

- Add the bananas to the blender. Let it sit in the blender for 2-3 minutes to soften slightly. Turn the blender on low and let it slowly chop up the fruit into small pieces.
- Add in the milk and blend, starting on low and working the speed up slowly, until smooth. Use a tamper or scrape down the sides as needed.
- Spoon the smoothie into a bowl and add on your desired toppings.

Nutrition per serving: calories 325kcal | protein 7g | carbs 57g | fat 10g | fiber 7g

181.   Blueberry Mango Smoothie Bowl

Preparation Time: 10 mins | Total Time: 10 mins | Servings: 1 serving
Ingredients:

- ¾ cup of frozen blueberries
- ¾ cup of frozen mango cubes
- ¾ cup of vanilla Greek yogurt nonfat
- ¾ cup of vanilla almond milk unsweetened Toppings (optional)
- 1 tsp cinnamon
- 1 tbsp. chia seeds
- 2 tbsps. granola
- 2 tbsps. chopped fruit (blueberries, strawberries, bananas)

Directions:

- Blend together frozen blueberries, mango, greek yogurt and almond milk. Blend until smooth.
- If smoothie does not mix smoothly, scrape down the sides, apply ¼ cup of almond milk and blend.
- Through a bowl. Top with preferred toppings. Eat promptly.

182.   Smoothie Bowl with Almond Milk, Banana, Spinach, and Almond Butter

Preparation Time: 5 minutes | Cooking Time: 0 minutes | Serving: 1
Ingredients:

- 1 large frozen banana
- 2 cups fresh spinach leaves
- 1/2 cup unsweetened almond milk
- 1 tablespoonful almond butter
- 1/4 cup sliced almonds for topping
- Optional toppings: fresh berries, shredded coconut, chia seeds, honey

Directions:

- Add the frozen banana, spinach, almond milk, and almond butter to a blender. Blend on high speed until smooth and creamy.

- Pour the smoothie into a bowl and sprinkle the sliced almonds on top.
- Add any additional toppings you like, such as fresh berries, shredded coconut, chia seeds, or a drizzle of honey.
- Serve and enjoy!

Nutrition per serving: Calories: 350 | Protein: 10g | Fat: 20g | Carbohydrates: 37g | Fiber: 8g | Sugar: 14g | Sodium: 175mg

183.   Muesli with Raspberries

Number of servings: 2
Ingredients:

- 1 cup muesli
- 1 ½ cups low-fat milk
- 2 cups raspberries

Directions:

- Divide muesli and raspberries into 2 bowls. Pour ¾ cup milk into each bowl and serve.

Nutrition per serving: Calories – 288 | Fat – 6.6 g | Carbohydrate – 51.8 g | Fiber – 13.3 g | Protein – 13 g

184.   Coconut Maple Walnut Granola

Prep Time: 5 Mins | Cook Time: 30 Mins | Total Time: 35 Minutes
Ingredients

- 2 cups of large flake oats (or rolled oats)
- ½ cup of chopped walnuts
- ½ cup of sliced almonds
- ¼ cup of chopped pecans
- ½ cup of pure maple syrup
- ¼ cup of melted coconut oil
- ½ tbsp vanilla extract
- 1 tsp ground cinnamon

Directions:

- Preheat the oven to 300 degrees Fahrenheit.
- Mix the barley, walnuts, almonds, and pecans in a big mixing bowl and whisk to mix.
- Mix the maple syrup, coconut oil, cocoa, and cinnamon in a medium mixing bowl. To mix, stir all together thoroughly.
- Pour the mixture into the big mixing bowl with the dry ingredients. Stir all together with a wooden spoon.
- Spread the granola mixture uniformly on a baking tray lined with aluminum foil or parchment paper.
- Preheat oven into 350°F and bake for 30 minutes. Take a tray out of the oven every 10 minute and give it a good stir. Replace the granola in the oven and re-spread it.
- Remove the granola from the oven and set aside to cool entirely.

185.   Mini Omelet Muffins

Number of servings: 2
Ingredients:

- 1–2 teaspoons olive oil
- ¼ cup skim milk or half and half
- 2 tablespoons grated cheddar cheese
- ½ cup chopped vegetables of your choice
- 1 teaspoon Italian seasoning

- 4 eggs
- Salt to taste

Directions:
- You need to preheat your oven to 350°F.
- As the oven is preheating, whisk eggs with milk, salt, and Italian seasoning.
- Stir in cheddar cheese and vegetables.
- Grease four ramekins with oil. Spoon the egg mixture into the ramekins.
- Place the ramekins in a baking pan. Pour hot water all around the ramekins, up to about ½ the height of the ramekin.
- Now place the ramekins along with the baking pan, in the oven and let it bake until it sets, about 30 minutes.
- You can also make the omelets in a muffin pan. Place the muffin pan directly in the oven

Nutrition per serving: Two muffins Calories: 370| Fat: 28 g| Carbohydrates: 3.2 g| Fiber: 2 g| Protein: 26 g

186.   Green Tea and Vanilla Ice Cream

Preparation time: 10min | Cooking time: 3h | Servings: 8
Ingredients:
- 1/2 (14.1-oz.) package refrigerated piecrusts (1 piecrust)
- 3 cups fresh figs, stemmed and quartered (about 15 oz.)
- 4 large eggs, beaten
- 3/4 cup granulated sugar
- 1/4 cup all-purpose flour
- 1/4 cup unsalted butter, melted
- 2 tablespoons fresh lemon juice (from 1 lemon)
- 2 teaspoons ground ginger
- Whipped cream

Directions:
- Preheat oven to 425°F. Fit piecrust into a 9- inch pie plate, pressing into bottom and up sides. Fold edges under, and crimp, if desired.
- Spread figs in an even layer in piecrust. Combine eggs, sugar, flour, butter, lemon juice, and ginger in a medium bowl, and stir vigorously until well blended. Pour over figs in piecrust.
- Bake on bottom rack of preheated oven for 10 minutes. Reduce temperature to 350°F; bake until center is set, about 40 minutes more. Cool completely on a wire rack, about 2 hours. Serve with whipped cream.

Nutrition per serving: calories 350kcal

187.   Bulgur Wheat with Dried Cranberries

Prep: 10 mins| Cook: 15 mins| Total: 25 mins| Yield: 2 servings
Ingredients
- 1 cup of water
- ½ cup of dry bulgur wheat
- 1 ½ tbsp. chicken bouillon granules
- 1 tsp butter
- ¼ cup of dried cranberries

Directions
- Bring the water to boil, then add the bulgur, bouillon granules, and butter. Cover bath, reduce heat to medium, and simmer.

- Add cooked bulgur and softly mix in the dried cranberries.

Nutrition per serving: 137 calories| protein 2.9g| carbohydrates 26.3g| fat 2.8g| cholesterol 6mg| sodium 864.9mg

188.   Chocolate Almond Pudding

Preparation time: 5 mins | Cook: 10 mins Total: 15 mins | Servings: 8 | Yield: 8 servings
Ingredients:
- ½ cup of sugar
- ⅓ cup of baking cocoa
- 2 tbsps. cornstarch
- 2 cups of milk
- 1 egg, beaten
- ¼ tsp vanilla extract
- ⅛ tsp almond extract

Directions:
- Mix together sugar, cocoa and cornstarch in a big saucepan. Add eggs and milk slowly. Cook on low heat for medium time until thickened. Take off heat and stir in vanilla and almond extracts. Garnish and serve.

Nutrition per serving: 104 calories| protein 3.5g| carbohydrates 19.2g| fat 2.3g| cholesterol 28.1mg| sodium 34.7mg.

189. Melon Mint Salad

Preparation Time: 10 Mins | Cook Time: 0 Mins | Total Time: 10 |Mins Yield: 6 Cups

Ingredients:
- 1 tbsp. honey
- 1 tbsp. lemon juice
- 6 cups of melon cubes
- ¼ cup of chopped fresh mint

Directions:
- Mix honey and lemon juice in one bowl.
- Stir in melon and mint.

Nutrition serving size: 1 cup of calories: 108.12 kcal | sugar: 25.27 g | carbohydrates: 26.47 g | fiber: 2.54 g | protein: 2.32 g

190. Seafood Salad with Lime Sauce

Preparation time: 15 minutes | Serves: 2

Ingredients:
- 4 Mussels, pieces
- 3 Cherry tomatoes
- 3 oz Cooked shrimp, shredded
- 2 oz Calamary
- 2 oz Iceberg lettuce
- 1/2 Lime
- 1.5 fl. oz Olive oil
- 1 oz. Pine nuts
- 1 tbsp. Cheese Parmesan, grated
- Pepper black ground, to taste

Directions:
- Boil the calamary and cut into strips. Tear lettuce leaves. Cherry tomatoes cut in half. Put the pine nuts on a dry frying pan and fry gently all the time
- Mix the juice of half lime with olive oil, add salt and black pepper to taste. Put all the ingredients on a plate and pour dressing. Sprinkle with pine nuts on top.

Nutrition per serving: Calories: 149 Kcal Fat: 12.2 g. | Protein: 8.1 g. | Carbs: 1.7 g

191. Sweet and Tangy Vinegar Coleslaw

Prep Time 20 minutes| Refrigerate 1 hour| Total Time 1 hour 20 minutes

Ingredients:
For the Crunchy Coleslaw
- 10 cups of shredded coleslaw mix or 1 16-ounce bag
- 1 cup of thinly sliced red onion
- 1 cup of shredded red cabbage
- 1 carrot thinly slivered
- 1/3 cup of canola oil
- 1/4 cup of apple cider vinegar
- 1 tbsp sugar
- 1 tsp caraway seeds
- 1 tsp celery seed
- 1 tsp kosher salt
- 1/2 tsp freshly ground black pepper

Directions:
- Mix the coleslaw blend, red onion, shredded red cabbage, and carrot in a big mixing bowl. Whisk the canola oil, apple cider vinegar, sugar, caraway seeds, celery seed, kosher salt, and freshly ground black pepper together in a shallow mixing bowl. Toss the cabbage mixture with the dressing. Cover and chills for 1 hour to allow flavors to meld.

192. Avocado Chicken Salad

Preparation Time: 15 minutes | Cooking Time: 0 minutes| Serving: 3

Ingredients:
For the Salad:
- 2 avocados, halved, peeled, pitted
- 1 cup shredded chicken
- ¼ teaspoon salt
- 4 hard-boiled eggs, peeled, chopped
- ¼ teaspoon ground black pepper
- ¼ cup sun-dried tomatoes, oil-packed, chopped
- ½ cup chopped basil and dill
- 2 tablespoons oil from sun-dried tomatoes
- ½ cup crumbled feta cheese
- 1 lemon, juiced

For Assembling:
- 6 slices of toasted whole-grain bread Arugula or microgreens, fresh, as needed

Directions:
- Prepare the salad and for this, take a medium bowl, place the avocado in it and then mash with a fork.
- Add tomatoes along with its oil, eggs, chicken, salt, herbs, lemon juice, and black pepper, and then stir until just mixed.
- Meal Prep: Divide the salad evenly among three meal prep containers, cover it tightly with plastic wrap so that there is no air, and then cover the containers with a lid.
- Store the containers in the refrigerator for up to 3 days and when ready to eat, bring the salad to room temperature. Toast the bread slices, spoon the salad evenly on three slices of toast, cover with microgreens, and then cover the top with remaining toasts. Serve straight away.

Nutrition per serving: Calories: 100 Cal| Total Fats: 100 g| Saturated Fat: 100 g| Carbohydrate: 100 g| Sugar: 100 g| Fiber: 100 g| Protein: 100 g

193. Salmon Couscous Salad

Number of servings: 2

Ingredients:
- ½ cup sliced cremini mushrooms
- 6 cups baby spinach
- ½ cup cooked whole wheat Israeli couscous
- ½ cup chopped, dried apricots
- ½ cup diced eggplant
- 8 ounces cooked salmon
- 1-ounce goat cheese, crumbled

For white wine vinaigrette:
- 4 tablespoons white wine vinegar
- Salt to taste
- Pepper to taste
- ½ cup extra-virgin olive oil

Directions:

- Place a skillet over medium heat. Spray some cooking spray into the skillet. Add eggplant and mushroom and cook until light brown and some of the cooked juices are visible. Turn off the heat.
- Place spinach in a bowl. Pour 2-3 tablespoons of the vinaigrette and toss well. Spread on a serving platter.
- Drizzle some vinaigrette over the couscous (as per your taste and store remaining vinegar if any in the refrigerator). Toss well.
- Spread couscous over the spinach. Next layer with salmon followed by cooked vegetables.
- Scatter apricots and goat cheese on top and serve

Nutrition per serving: Four cups Calories: 464| Fat: 22.1 g| Carbohydrates: 34.7 g| Fiber: 5.9 g| Protein: 34.8 g

194.   Celery Citrus Salad

Ingredients
- 5 tangerines or mandarin oranges
- ¼ cup of feta cheese
- 2 tbsps. golden balsamic vinegar
- 1 cup of roughly chopped celery leaves
- 2 cups of sliced celery
- 4 cups of (approximately ¼ pound) mixed salad greens
- ½ cup of chopped pecans
- Cracked black pepper

Dedication:
- Squeeze one of the fruits into a large bowl. Add the vinegar and cheese and combine them well with a fork.
- Peel the remaining fruit and cut any stringy pieces before adding them to the bowl.
- Remove tomatoes, sliced onion, and lettuce, and toss well. Cover with pecans and add black pepper as need.

195.   Tuna Salad

Preparation time: 5 min | Cooking time: 0 min | Servings: 6
Ingredients:
- 4 (5 ounce) cans tuna packed in water drained (see note 1)
- 1 cup mayonnaise or less to taste (see note 2)
- 1/3 cup celery finely chopped (about 1 rib)
- 2 tablespoons red onion minced, about 2 small slices
- 2 tablespoons sweet pickle relish (see note 3)
- 1 tablespoon fresh lemon juice
- 1 clove garlic minced
- salt and freshly ground black pepper

Directions:
- In a medium bowl, combine tuna, mayonnaise, celery, onion, relish, lemon juice, and garlic. -Season to taste with salt and pepper (I like ½ teaspoons salt and ¼ teaspoon pepper). Serve immediately or cover and chill until serving.

Nutrition per serving: calories 345kcal | protein 11g | carbs 3g | fat 1g | fiber 1g

196.   Vibrant Raspberry Walnut Salad

Preparation Time: 10 minutes| Cook Time: 0 minutes
Ingredients:
- 3 cups of kale
- 1 cucumber chopped
- 1 cup of raspberries
- 1/2 cup of walnuts chopped
- 1/4 cup of sunflower seeds
- 2 tbsp crumbled feta

Directions:
- For this salad, we like to coarsely chop the kale in a food processor, although this step is optional. You may just use torn/chopped or baby kale leaves as is if you like. In the large mixing bowl, combine the chopped kale and the mayonnaise.
- Toss the salad with cucumber, raspberries, walnuts, sunflower seeds, and feta. To mix is to mingle
- Drizzle with your favorite olive oil-based dressing. This recipe for Simple Lemon Vinaigrette is one of our favorites.

197.   Southern-Style Potato Salad

Prep Time: 10 mins | Cooking Time: 4 mins | Number of Servings: 2
Ingredients:
- 4 medium Russet potatoes, peeled and cubed
- 2 eggs1 celery stalk, chopped
- ¼ red onion, chopped
- ¼ cup plain Greek yogurt
- 2 tablespoons yellow mustard
- Kosher salt
- Freshly ground black pepper
- Paprika, for garnish

Directions:
- Put 1 cup of water and the potatoes into the cooker pot. Put the whole eggs (in their shells) on top of the potatoes.
- Secure the lid and cook on high pressure for 4 minutes. Use a quick release at the end of the cooking time. Remove the lid and take out the eggs. Carefully remove the cooker pot, then drain the potatoes through a large sieve or colander and set aside.
- Rinse the eggs under cold water until they are no longer steaming. Place them into a bowl of cold water to chill. When cooled, peel and roughly chop them.
- In a medium bowl, combine the potatoes, eggs, celery, onion, yogurt, and mustard, then season with salt and pepper.
- Transfer the potato salad to a serving bowl, sprinkle with paprika, and cover and refrigerate until ready to serve.

Nutrition per serving: Calories: 397| Total fat: 6g| Saturated fat: 2g| Cholesterol: 167mg| Carbohydrates: 71g| Fiber: 11g| Protein: 17g

198.   Mediterranean Tuna Salad with No Mayo!

Ingredients:
- 2 cans Genova Seafood Yellowfin Tuna
- 1 cucumber, chopped
- 1/2 red onion, diced
- 1 cup of roasted red peppers, chopped
- 1/2 cup of pepperocini, diced
- 1/3 cup of parsley, finely chopped
- Sundried tomatoes, chopped

- 2 tsp capers
- Optional: 1/4 cup of feta cheese
- Optional olive
- Optional: 1 14.5 ounces can chickpeas, drained and rinsed
- 1/2 avocado, diced
- Pinch of fine sea salts
- Pinch of black pepper

Red Wine Vinaigrette:
- 2 tbsp olive oil
- 2 tbsp red wine vinegar
- 1 tsp lemon juice
- 1 tsp dried parsley
- 1 tsp dried oregano
- Pinch fine salt
- Pinch black pepper

Dedication:
- Combine all of the salad ingredients in a large mixing bowl.
- Whisk together a dressing ingredients in a small bowl.
- Toss the ingredients in the dressing to combine.
- Taste and adjust the seasonings as needed!
- Serve over a salad, over a sandwich, with spaghetti, lettuce wraps, or half an avocado!

199. Roasted Broccoli Salad

Total: 30 min Active: 15 min | Yield: 4 servings

Ingredients
- ¼ cup of olive oil
- 2 bunches broccoli, florets separated
- 1 red onion, halved and thinly sliced
- Kosher salt and freshly ground black pepper
- 4 slices thick-cut bacon
- ½ cup of sour cream
- ¼ cup of mayonnaise
- 3 tbsps. whole milk
- 1 tsp granulated sugar
- 1 tsp paprika
- 3 tbsps. chopped fresh parsley

Directions

- Heat the oven to 425 F.
- Toss the broccoli florets, red onion, olive oil, salt and pepper in a medium dish. Roast the broccoli, flipping halfway around, until the sides are crispy, 18 to 20 mins. Cool, then transfer to a bowl.
- In a skillet, cook all the bacon until it's crisp, 12 to 14 mins. Set back.
- Mix sour cream, mayonnaise and milk together in a little bowl. Season with cinnamon, paprika, 1 tbsp minced parsley, 2 tsp salt and a pinch of pepper.
- Add the bacon and parsley to the cooled broccoli, then coat with enough dressing to coat and blend. Add the remaining chopped parsley.

To make ahead, assemble the salad, refrigerate

200. Chickpea Avocado Salad

Prep Time: 8-10 mins | Cooking Time: 12 mins | Number of Servings: 2

Ingredients:
- 1/4 cup avocado, chopped
- 2 tablespoons pomegranate seeds
- 1 cup chickpeas, soaked and rinsed
- 1/2 cup quinoa
- 1 teaspoon rice vinegar

Directions:
- Turn on the heat, add the chickpea in a pot and 1 cup water and Stir the ingredients to combine well. The close the pot
- Pressure will slowly build up; let the added ingredients cook
- Drain water and set aside chickpea.
- Add the quinoa and 1/2 cup water in the cooking pot. Stir the ingredients to combine well. Then close the pot.
- Drain and add quinoa with the chickpea. Add the vinegar, pomegranate, and avocado on top; serve.

Nutritional Values (Per Serving): Calories – 566| Fat – 12g| Carbohydrates – 26g| Fiber – 12g| Sodium – 62mg| Protein – 25g

	Breakfast	Lunch	Dinner
Day 1	Eggs with Zucchini Noodles	Mushroom Risotto	Seafood Couscous Paella
Day 2	Mixed Berry Oatmeal	Cabbage with Shrimps and Lemongrass	Chicken Lettuce Wraps
Day 3	Baked Eggs with Pesto	Balsamic Roasted Carrots and Baby Onions	Salmon with Sorrel Sauce
Day 4	Fried Eggs with Smoked Salmon and Lemon Cream	Greek Meatballs	Baked Clams Oreganata
Day 5	Indian Masala Omelet Recipe	Broccoli-Cheddar Scalloped Potatoes	Canapes with Cheese, Tomato, and Salmon
Day 6	Shrimp, Avocado & Feta Wrap	Herby Fish with Wilted Greens & Mushrooms	Grilled Chicken Caesar Salad with Whole Grain Croutons
Day 7	Avocado Toast with Poached Egg and Cherry Tomatoes	Vegetable Frittata	Italian Artichoke and Green Bean Casserole
Day 8	Blueberry Mango Smoothie Bowl	Baked Cod and Veggies	White Bean Soup
Day 9	Scrambled Eggs with Bell Peppers, Onions, and Cheddar Cheese	Balsamic Pork and Strawberry Salad	Hot Sandwiches with Cheese, Tomatoes and Greens
Day 10	Fried Eggs in Bread	Fish Stew with Potatoes and Tomatoes	Slow-Cooker Quinoa with Arugula
Day 11	Tomato-Basil Consommé	Pasta with Asparagus	Southern-Style Potato Salad
Day 12	Pita Pizza	Cherry Tomato Salad with Shrimps	Roasted Broccoli Salad
Day 13	Mediterranean Tofu Scramble	Pork Stir Fry	Fava Beans with Jasmine Rice Recipe
Day 14	Ham 'N Cheese Scrambled Eggs	Mediterranean Fish Skillet	Black Bean-Quinoa Buddha Bowl
Day 15	Oatmeal with Sun-Dried Tomato and Parmesan Cheese	Crockpot Chicken Tacos	Seafood Gumbo
Day 16	Blueberry Coffee Breakfast Smoothie	Cacio e Pepe Spaghetti Squash	Southern Beans and Greens
Day 17	Apple Pancakes (Breakfast)	Eggplant in Sesame	Dilly Salmon

Day 18	Veggie Omelet with Bell Peppers, Onions, and Goat Cheese	Spanakopita	Cabbage with Shrimps and Lemongrass
Day 19	Crustless Tuna Breakfast Quiche	Mediterranean Chicken Quinoa Bowl	Charred Shrimp, Pesto & Quinoa Bowls
Day 20	Scrambled Eggs with Whole Grain Toast and Sliced Avocado	Easy Sautéed Kale	Curried Tilapia Brown Rice Bowl
Day 21	Cauliflower Tabbouleh with Chicken	Skillet Salmon with Tomato Quinoa	Ravioli & Vegetable Soup
Day 22	Mediterranean Breakfast Board	Grilled Lamb Chops with a Side of Chickpeas and Sautéed Spinach	Lemon Salmon with Garlic and Thyme
Day 23	Breakfast Granola	Spinach & Bean Burrito Wrap	Roasted Fish with Vegetables
Day 24	Banana smoothie bowl	Veggie Omelet	Mediterranean Plant Protein Power Bowl
Day 25	Avocado Breakfast Scramble	Oatmeal Pancakes	Pork Rinds Crusted Salmon Patties | Gluten-Free | Nut-Free
Day 26	Banana, Raisin, and Walnut Baked Oatmeal	Pot Roast with Winter Root Vegetables	Spicy Cauliflower Rice with Ground Turkey
Day 27	Cheesy Broccoli and Cauliflower Broth	Slow Cooker Beef Bourguignon	Grilled Squid
Day 28	Berry Chia Pudding	Swift Fried Rice	Creamy Salmon Soup
Day 29	Banana Bread Smoothie	Lentil Soup	Oven-Poached Lemon Butter Cod
Day 30	Eggs with Zucchini Noodles	Kidney Bean Curry	Spiced Beef Pilaf

As we come to the close of "200 Mediterranean Recipes", I hope you've found more than just a collection of dishes. Within these pages lies a journey through sun-kissed landscapes, bustling marketplaces, and intimate family dinners. Each recipe carries with it a story, a tradition, and a taste of the rich Mediterranean heritage.

The 30-day meal plan is designed not only to guide you through a month of wholesome eating but also to immerse you in a lifestyle that cherishes food as a communal experience, one that nourishes the body, warms the heart, and binds us together.

As you venture into your kitchen, armed with these recipes, remember that cooking is an act of love. Whether you're preparing a quick snack or a grand feast, you're partaking in a tradition that has been passed down through generations.

Thank you for letting this book be a part of your culinary journey. Here's to vibrant health, memorable meals, and the simple joy of cooking. Enjoy every bite, and as they say around the Mediterranean table, "Sahtain!" - May it be good for your soul and health.

www.ingramcontent.com/pod-product-compliance
Lightning Source LLC
Chambersburg PA
CBHW080425030426
42335CB00020B/2596